"What on earth made you think I was a GP?"

Now she seemed to be burning from the inside out as she realized she might have gotten this whole scenario wrong. "The clinic..."

"Well, unless you have four legs or wings, you're not likely to be one of my patients, I'm afraid. I'm the local vet. I'm sorry if you thought otherwise."

The bell of shame was ringing loudly in her ears. She'd just bared her soul to a complete stranger because she'd assumed it was a confidential conversation, with a medical professional! Someone who worked in human medicine, at least.

Now it was apparent she'd simply humiliated herself in front of one of her new neighbors. Worse...

"Is this the Loch Bruce Veterinary Practice?" she asked, her soul about to leave her body.

"Yes. Why?"

"You're my new boss..."

Dear Reader,

I spend a lot of time in Scotland. It's one of my favorite places to be. This year we found a quiet loch, which seemed the ideal place for a country vet to hide away from the world. The tranquillity there also provided the perfect backdrop for my heroine to start her new life, away from the city.

Eloise and Daniel are an older couple, but hopefully their story will prove that it's never too late to find love. Sometimes there's even a second chance to have it when you think that part of your life is over.

I hope you enjoy their story as much as I enjoyed writing it.

Karin xx

TEMPTED BY HER OFF-LIMITS BOSS

KARIN BAINE

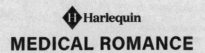

MEDICAL ROMANCE

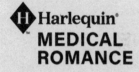

Harlequin®
MEDICAL ROMANCE

ISBN-13: 978-1-335-94296-8

Tempted by Her Off-Limits Boss

Copyright © 2025 by Karin Baine

Harlequin Enterprises ULC
22 Adelaide St. West, 41st Floor
Toronto, Ontario M5H 4E3, Canada
www.Harlequin.com

Printed in U.S.A.

Recycling programs for this product may not exist in your area.

Karin Baine lives in Northern Ireland with her husband, two sons and her out-of-control notebook collection. Her mother and her grandmother's vast collection of books inspired her love of reading and her dream of becoming a Harlequin author. Now she can tell people she has a *proper* job! You can follow Karin on X @karinbaine1 or visit her website for the latest news, karinbaine.com.

Books by Karin Baine

Harlequin Medical Romance

Carey Cove Midwives

Festive Fling to Forever

Christmas North and South

Festive Fling with the Surgeon

Royal Docs

Surgeon Prince's Fake Fiancée
A Mother for His Little Princess

A GP to Steal His Heart
Single Dad for the Heart Doctor
Falling Again for the Surgeon
Nurse's Risk with the Rebel
An American Doctor in Ireland
Midwife's One-Night Baby Surprise
Nurse's New Year with the Billionaire

Visit the Author Profile page
at Harlequin.com for more titles.

For my own older hero xx

CHAPTER ONE

ELOISE CARTER WAS in the middle of nowhere. Nothing but darkness lay ahead. Of course, that was exactly why she was moving to the village of Bruce Valley in Ayrshire for peace and quiet. Though she hadn't counted on driving up this narrow, twisted lane in the pitch dark *en route* to her new home next to Loch Bruce, not realising there were no streetlights

With no Internet signal, she couldn't get the sat nav to direct her either. The stress was making her blood pressure rise—something she didn't need when peri-menopause was already wreaking havoc inside her. She switched on the air conditioning as her body temperature went into overdrive despite the cool night. Another lovely symptom of being almost fifty years old was a completely banjaxed internal thermostat.

'This is hopeless!' She hit the steering wheel in temper, when leaning closer to the windscreen didn't prove useful.

Suddenly, she was blinded by the glare of headlights as another vehicle came straight for her. She swung the car to the right and into a shallow ditch, narrowly missing a head-on collision. Hyperventilating, gripping onto the steering wheel so hard her knuckles were white, she sat stunned in the driver seat, realising her new life had almost been over before it began.

This move from Glasgow was supposed to be her new start, a shift away from all the bad things in her life. She'd only left the city a matter of hours ago and she'd already nearly got herself killed.

Someone rapped on the window and she nearly jumped out of her skin. 'Are you okay?'

She wound down the window, not about to open the door to a strange man in the middle of nowhere. 'I'm fine.'

'You're going to have trouble getting out of that ditch. Let me help you.'

'I said I'm fine. Now, leave me alone.' She couldn't quite see the man who'd almost run her off the road, but he was backlit by the high beam still blazing in the darkness, and it was obvious he was tall and broad. Despite Eloise's apparently ever-expanding waist these days, she would still be no match for him.

'I'm not going to leave you out here all by

yourself…' He was persistent, and did nothing to assuage her anxiety.

Ignoring him, Eloise stuck the car into reverse and put her foot down, succeeding only in making a lot of noise and polluting the air with exhaust fumes as the car refused to move. It was hardly surprising when it had been overloaded with all of her belongings. Her entire life was packed into the ancient black car.

'You might need to lose some of the weight bogging your car down,' he suggested with a sigh.

'I know that *now*.' Eloise bristled as she undid her seatbelt. She had no choice but to get out or she'd be stuck here all night. All she could do was hope that, since he sounded more ticked off than she was right now, it meant he wasn't some psycho serial-killer. Not that it excused his terrible driving, which had forced her off the road in the first place.

'This is your fault, you know. If you hadn't been hogging the road, I wouldn't have had to take evasive action,' she griped, as she got out of the car and began untying the large canvas bag attached to the roof of the car, which contained most of her clothes.

'I wasn't expecting anyone else to be out here

at this time of night. I was on my way back from an emergency call. Sorry.'

The tall, dark stranger sounded apologetic and helped her undo the straps attaching her luggage to the car. If he'd been out on a call it suggested he was part of the emergency services—a doctor, perhaps, someone she could trust, though she wasn't going to satisfy him by asking what he did. This wasn't a social event. Eloise just needed to get her car back on the road so she could get to her new home and hopefully she'd find something in her belongings that would constitute dinner.

Today had been a whirlwind trying to get the car packed and saying all her goodbyes at work, then she'd got caught in the city rush-hour traffic. She'd expected to get here earlier.

Actually, she'd hoped to be here days ago, since she was supposed to be starting her new job in the morning, but they'd been short staffed at the veterinary clinic where she worked as a nurse. Soft touch that she was, she'd agreed to stay on to relieve some of the pressure. That meant leaving herself short on time. She hadn't even stopped for anything to eat and, though she could stand to lose a few pounds, she needed some sustenance when she was already feeling a little lightheaded.

Once her roadside assistant had heaved the heavy bag to one side, Eloise got back into the car and tried again to manoeuvre it out of the ditch. There came more revving, wheel spinning, clutch burning, swearing and not much else.

'OK, stop, before you dig yourself in completely.' The stranger tapped on the roof to get her to stop.

Eloise just about managed to hold in a scream as she got out again for another look at her predicament. Whether she got out of her seat too quickly, or the uneven earth knocked her off-balance, she had a little wobble. A little lightheaded, she fought hard to regain her composure.

Strong hands caught her around the waist and steadied her. 'Are you okay?'

'Yes,' she insisted, brushing away any offer of help.

This past year and a half she'd had no choice but to do everything on her own, and she certainly didn't need outside interference now from someone she didn't know. With her girls having flown the nest to start their own lives, and her husband, Sam, doing the same—deciding he didn't love her enough to stick around after thirty years—she hadn't had much choice but to go it alone.

The breakdown of her marriage had come as a shock at the time, as she'd believed they were comfortable and happy, if not as in love as they had been in the beginning, but she'd had time to come to terms with it. And the fact she'd probably be on her own for the rest of her days. She couldn't imagine putting all that time and effort into another relationship only to have it thrown back in her face when she needed support more than ever.

A mishap with her car wasn't going to be the end of the world compared to all she'd gone through. Except, when she stepped away from him, her head began to spin again, her skin felt flushed and she suddenly felt very clammy. She stumbled, fighting the darkness which was threatening to close in.

'I've got you.' There were those big arms around her again, catching her, saving her from collapsing onto the ground.

And, oh, he smells so good...

'I said, I don't need your help,' she grumbled, though made no attempt to push him away this time.

'I know, but humour me.' She could hear the smile in his voice. 'Why don't I take you back to my clinic and make you some sweet tea? I'll make a few calls and get someone to pull your car out.'

'I just haven't had anything to eat today. It's probably my blood sugar…' She really should have known better; she'd have to start taking better care of herself. No one else was going to do it.

'Well, I'm sure I can find you a snack at my office.' The stranger guided her to his car and, though she probably should have resisted, there was something about him that made Eloise feel safe. Perhaps it was his calm demeanour, or the mention of his clinic—it could even have been the promise of snacks—but she trusted him and went with him willingly.

'Is there anyone I can call for you?' Daniel was desperate to hand over responsibility for this woman to someone else. The last thing he wanted was to bring her back to his practice out of surgery hours without his receptionist to run interference.

As well as his business, it was his home, and he wasn't used to sharing that part of his life any more—not since he'd lost Anne five years ago. She'd been his soul mate, the only person who'd understood him. Without her he'd regressed back to the person he'd been before she'd barged into his life: a loner who only associated with the outside world when he had to. Though the nature of his job made that unavoidable, he did at least have control over who did, or didn't, come into his home at night… until now.

However, it was his fault she'd ended up on the side of the road and he couldn't leave her here alone. He hadn't taken as much care as he should have on his way home, not expecting to meet any other traffic. There were so few people who lived this far out, most of them at an age when they didn't venture out after dark, so he hadn't imagined seeing anyone else. He should've known better, and was lucky there hadn't been a more serious incident.

'There's no one. I've just moved here from Glasgow. Hence the overloaded car…' His passenger settled herself in his car as he tied her bag to the roof and got in next to her.

'Ah. I heard someone had bought the old place near the loch. It's going to be quite the change of pace, moving here from the big city.'

'That's what I'm hoping,' she mumbled, staring out of the window into the darkness.

'Is your family joining you?' It wasn't any of his business, and if he was honest he wasn't really interested; he was just trying to make small talk, something he had to do a lot of during clinic appointments.

She shook her head, apparently not wishing to divulge any further personal information. That was fine by him. As soon as he was sure she was okay to send on her merry way again, he'd be washing his hands of this spiky stranger. He was glad when they finally pulled up outside the surgery to end the awkwardness of the situation.

'Well, this is us. I'll get you settled with something to eat and drink and make a couple of calls.' Then hopefully he could lock the door on the outside world again.

Eloise sat down with a heavy sigh once her host had illuminated his small office with bright fluorescent light. She felt a little safer, knowing he was a medical professional and not just some opportunist murderer who'd got her to come with him under false pretences. In a village this small, the likelihood was that he'd end up being her local GP anyway, so she should probably stop being so defensive around him. She was going to need his assistance for the foreseeable future for all the joys which came with being an older woman.

'I'll just go and make us some tea. Make yourself, er, comfortable.'

He disappeared out through the door again, leaving her to take in the sparse surroundings of brilliant white walls, a couple of chairs and laptop on the desk. It didn't exactly scream, 'homely, village doc'. Some doctors she knew liked to decorate their work space with a few personal mementos to give the room some personality: a family photo, a whimsical mug, or an inspirational quote on the wall. Not so here; she couldn't get a feel of the man at all.

Although, now she'd seen him in the light, she could tell he was handsome. His black hair was threaded heavily with strands of silver, and long dark lashes framed his deep-brown eyes. He had an outdoors tan and broad shoulders which tapered down into a narrow waist. She was sure more than a couple of his patients must harbour a crush on the doctor, especially given his sympathetic bedside manner.

The opposite sex hadn't held much interest for her since the divorce, or the realisation that she was apparently past her prime—invisible to most, now that she was approaching fifty, and apparently holding no appeal for any man, including her husband. That didn't mean she couldn't appreciate a handsome older man. This one was striking and very much in his prime.

He came back in clutching two steaming mugs of tea and handed one to her, before taking the seat opposite. Their knees almost touching created an intimacy between them which made Eloise's pulse flutter.

'How are you feeling now?' he asked, presenting her with a chocolate-covered, caramel wafer biscuit.

Her rumbling stomach, and need for a sugar rush, bypassed the usual polite refusal in response. She unwrapped it and savoured the sweet treat as he finished his in two bites.

'Better now,' she finally offered. Though it wasn't strictly true. Perhaps in all the chaos to get here she'd been avoiding all of the issues which had weighed her down lately and, although this little interlude was giving her body a boost, her mind was just as burdened as ever.

'Really?' He cocked a dark eyebrow, seemingly not fooled by her pretence. The sign of a good doctor, she supposed, who could see beyond the façade and was willing to take the time to discover the truth—vital in getting to the heart of what ailed his patients.

She supposed there was no harm in being honest. It might do her good to get some stuff off her chest, and he might be able to help her move forward in this new chapter of her life.

'No. Not really.' She leaned back into her chair with a sigh, as though the weight on her shoulders of having to keep it together had finally been lifted. This felt like a safe space, somewhere she could actually open up about everything.

Besides, by pouring out her heart to him, she'd absolutely have to ditch any romantic notions towards this man. It would be a strictly doctor-patient relationship in the future. There'd be nothing romantic about a middle-aged woman having an emotional breakdown in his office, and she'd only embarrass herself to think otherwise.

Eloise took a sip of the sweet tea and the floodgates seemed to open.

'I'm a forty-nine-year-old woman who's perimenopausal. My husband has just divorced me rather than stick around to support me, or "waste any more of my life with someone I don't really love".' She couldn't help the accompanying tut and eye-roll.

It seemed like such a ridiculous thing to say after thirty years of marriage. It was as if it meant nothing to him, and their whole time together had been a sham. They'd had some good times together, and Eloise had imagined they'd have some more. Apparently her husband had other ideas. It had left her feeling worthless, a burden, surplus to requirements. She didn't know how she was ever going to get past that, knowing she no longer had a place in the world as a wife or mother. No one needed her any more and, after having looked after others for half of her life, she didn't know what to do with her life now.

'I'm sorry.' The doctor frowned and she was convinced he genuinely empathised with her situation, given he probably dealt with this story every day of his working week: middle-aged women who'd outlived their usefulness being nursemaid, cleaner and cook suddenly finding themselves on the scrapheap for the crime of getting older.

'It's not your fault, is it?' She flashed him a wobbly smile. It wasn't hers either, but her ex had firmly laid all the blame for their marriage ending at her door, taking no responsibility or making any effort to save it.

'Perhaps you're better off without him.' Daniel shrugged.

'Oh, I know I am now, it just took a while to get used to the idea. But it's not just about that... I suppose it's the end of my life as I know it. My girls have both moved out, I've left my job and my home I've had for decades, never mind what my poor body is going through: insomnia, sweating, bloating, never knowing when my period's coming or how long it's going to last for. It's no wonder my husband doesn't find me attractive. I revolt myself these days.'

She gave a brittle laugh, because all of it was true. Out of the blue, her comfortable, predictable life had suddenly been turned on its head, and there was nothing she could rely on these days, not even her own body.

He cleared his throat. Eloise knew she was over-sharing, but he was a doctor, he could take it, and he was going to know what he was dealing with sooner or later. She was a mess and she was going to need his help to manage this next stage of her life.

'I'm sure you'll get through it.'

It seemed an odd thing for a doctor to say, not offering any solution or counselling. She didn't know what she'd been hoping for other than sharing her burden, but she was sure it was more than that. He hadn't struck her as the kind of doctor who'd tell her she was making a lot of fuss over nothing, but he wasn't giving her any practical advice on how to deal with her physical ailments at least.

'Is this it, then?'

He looked at her in bewilderment. 'Pardon me?'

'Is this just going to be my life for ever now—an endless round of unpleasant symptoms I have to put up with until eventually I turn into a dried-up old hag?'

A touch overdramatic? Perhaps. But that was how it felt these days—that she had no hope, or prospects, other than eventually her womanhood would completely be taken away from her. It would be nature reminding her that she was well past her 'best before' date. As though she was in any doubt.

'I'm sure it must feel like that now, but it won't last for ever. There are different things you can take to ease the symptoms. My wife went through it all too, and I know how rough it was for her. You have my sympathies.'

His affirmation that this wasn't all in her head was appreciated. She found herself looking at his ring finger for signs that he hadn't just made up a wife in order to sympathise with her. Although there was no glinting gold band to signify that he was indeed taken, there was a telltale pale ring of skin around his finger to suggest he had been married once upon a time. Eloise couldn't help but wonder if that was the point at which his married life had ended too. Had he been unable and unwilling to cope with his partner's physical changes, and sought a new life away from her? She suddenly found she no longer wanted his sympathies if he hadn't been able to extend them to his poor wife when she'd needed them.

'I had hoped for something more than your sympathy, like hormones, or whatever it is you usually prescribe...' With everything that had been going on at home, she'd put a lot of her medical issues down to stress, but she couldn't ignore the fact any longer that her body was changing and she would accept whatever help was out there.

'I'm not sure you'll want the usual hormones we prescribe here.' His hearty laugh was out of keeping with her impression of the caring local GP, as well as their current conversation.

'What do you mean? You're the doctor here. I thought that was what's recommended for women going through menopause.'

Eloise was beginning to think they were having two very different conversations here. Especially when he wore a puzzled frown in response. 'I'm not sure what that has to do with me.'

'You're a GP. Given the size of this town, I

assume you're soon to become my GP. Okay, so I haven't officially joined the practice yet, but I would've thought you'd take some interest in a potential patient.' All the stress was beginning to build up inside her again, as she'd apparently opened up to someone who had no interest in her problems.

'What on earth made you think I was a GP?'

Now she seemed to burn from the inside out as she realised she might have got this whole scenario wrong. 'The clinic…'

'Well, unless you have four legs or wings, you're not likely to be one of my patients, I'm afraid. I'm the local vet. I'm sorry if you thought otherwise.'

The bell of shame rang loudly in her ears. She'd just bared her soul to a complete stranger because she'd assumed it was a confidential conversation with a medical professional! Someone who worked in human medicine, at least.

Now it was apparent she'd simply humiliated herself in front of one of her new neighbours… and worse…

'Is this the Loch Bruce Veterinary Practice?' she asked, her soul about to leave her body.

'Yes. Why?'

'You're my new boss…'

CHAPTER TWO

DANIEL WAS ON tenterhooks waiting for his new employee to arrive, so he could only imagine how she would feel after their unfortunate introduction last night. The misunderstanding over his job, which had caused her a great deal of embarrassment, had been entirely down to her, though perhaps he should have interrupted when she'd shared such deeply personal information, should have realised something was amiss. He'd simply assumed she needed to get her problems off her chest and he'd provided a listening ear. It was clear she'd been through a lot, and he'd never intended to make life even more difficult for her, but they'd got off to a very shaky start.

He didn't know which of them would be more embarrassed to see the other this morning. Actually, he did, and he was sorry her start here would be on a sour note. His concerns were affirmed when she turned up at the main entrance looking rather sheepish.

'Hi.' She was biting her lip, her pale-blue eyes fixed on him, probably waiting for him to address last night.

'Hi. Come in, come in. The others shouldn't be long.' Daniel was hoping Brooke, his receptionist, and Debbie, his fellow vet, wouldn't be too far behind to welcome her. She might feel more comfortable with others around to break the tension between them.

It was probably that need to keep some sort of barrier between the outside world and him which had caused the confusion in the first place. He'd left it to the other members of staff to hire his replacement nurse. If he'd done the job himself, he'd have known exactly who he was dealing with last night and vice versa.

'I'm Daniel Grant.' He introduced himself to the curvy brunette—a little too late, as it turned out.

'Eloise Carter. Can we talk about last night?' She got straight to the point, which he appreciated. After the misunderstanding last night, she'd left in such a hurry there hadn't been much opportunity to apologise.

'Of course.' He led her into his office and could see her cringe at the memory of everything she'd shared with him in that room only a matter of hours ago.

'I take it Gary got you sorted out last night?'

'Thank you for the tea and arranging help to recover my car.'

They stumbled over each other's words, then exchanged embarrassed grins. It was going to be difficult working together if it continued to be so toe-curling and awkward between them.

'Gary was a great help, thanks.'

Daniel had wondered if she'd got home okay, but she'd fled the building the minute the local farmer had arrived with his tractor to help tow her car. Daniel had considered phoning her, certain that he would've found her contact number on her job application form if he'd bothered to look at it. In the end, he'd thought it best to give Eloise some space from him to recover.

'And is everything okay with the house?' Here they were, back to making small talk, but he was reluctant to be the first to confront the elephant in the room.

'Yes. It'll take some work, and I still have to unpack everything, but I'll get there eventually.'

'Good. Good.' He nodded, and spent a long time staring down at his shoes.

'Look, I know last night wasn't your fault…'

'A misunderstanding.'

'Yes, well, it's all very embarrassing for me to have poured my heart out to you. Especially given that I'm going to be working for you for the foreseeable future.' She was clutching her bag and coat so tightly, he worried she might run out again and cancel the whole job contract.

'All forgotten, and I promise I won't say a word to anyone.' That was all he could do. They couldn't change what had happened and he couldn't unhear her troubles. Nor, he supposed, would he forget everything she'd confided in him, but he could assure her it wouldn't go any further.

'Thank you. It would be great if we could just put it behind us.'

'Done,' he said, with a clap of his hands. He hoped that they could start over as work colleagues, with Eloise as his new employee he knew nothing about. Except deep down he knew it was going to be impossible to forget the strength it must have taken this incredible woman to pick herself up and move here on her own to start again. Goodness knew he hadn't managed to do it in five years.

'Ah, the rest of the team are here. Let me make the introductions.' Daniel seemed as relieved as she was to hear the sound of other people in the building, opening the door to usher them both back out into the public domain.

It hadn't been easy, coming in to face him this morning, and sleep last night had proved impossible. She didn't think she'd ever get over the humiliation, and had spent most of the time since her outburst recounting every very personal detail she'd shared with her new boss. The best she could hope for was that they'd both pretend it had never happened, and that he wouldn't think it was some amusing anecdote he could trot out at parties. The disaster which was her personal life was not for dinner conversation, and something she wouldn't have shared at all if she hadn't been convinced he was a doctor.

'Hi.' She waved nervously at the two young blondes who'd walked in together.

'This is Debs and Brooke, and this is Eloise, our new recruit.' Daniel made the introductions, though they weren't strictly necessary, since they were the ones who'd done the interview process with her over numerous video calls.

'Hello again.' Debbie and Brooke stepped forward to shake her hand.

Eloise was able to relax a little, seeing some familiar faces. They'd hit it off immediately when they'd spoken before, despite the twenty-year age gap. However, she couldn't help but think that if Daniel had been more involved in the recruitment process, rather than delegating the responsibility to other members of staff, then they might've avoided her complete humiliation last night.

'It's good to finally meet you in person,' Eloise said, genuinely meaning it.

The enthusiasm and camaraderie which had been apparent from these two had been enough to convince her once and for all to pack up what was left of her life and move here. Again, if Daniel had done the interview himself, the outcome might have been very different.

'I'll let you get acquainted and show Eloise around while I get ready for the clinic.' Daniel didn't bother waiting around for anyone to agree. It was clear who was boss around here. It helped her breathe a little easier when he disappeared back into his office, out of sight.

'You know, he's not what I expected…' Eloise ruminated aloud, watching him walk away. From the way they'd spoken about the surgery owner, she'd imagined him to be some old man, out of touch and relying heavily on the youth of his staff. Although there was an age difference, Daniel was not some past-it old fogey— far from it.

'Pay no mind to him. Daniel prefers the company of animals to people.' Debbie had clearly misunderstood her comment, thinking she was in some way disappointed.

Concerned was the word she'd be most likely to use. She'd been expecting someone on the brink of retirement, perhaps leaving the running of the place to the youngsters, not a handsome older, very capable man. She realised she'd been using the word handsome a lot to describe Daniel in her head, and that alone was a warning sign. Uprooting and coming here hadn't been about rediscovering an interest in the opposite sex, especially in another troubled divorcee, and her boss. Hopefully it was a passing phase and she'd get over the fact he was good-looking soon enough.

'What about his family?' she found herself asking, despite telling herself his personal life was none of her business. It would help her better understand the man she was working with, she told herself. And, since she'd spilled her guts about her background, it seemed only fair she should know something about him too. Perhaps then she wouldn't feel quite so much as if she was starting here on the back foot.

'He doesn't have any. At least, none of his own, and I've never known of any other relatives. Other than Anne, of course.' Debbie dropped her head as though it was a subject she shouldn't be talking about, which only increased Eloise's curiosity.

'Anne… Is that his wife?'

Both women nodded solemnly.

'I never knew her,' the receptionist was quick to point out.

'And I started after she'd gone,' Debbie added.

'Gone?' There was obviously some sort of scandal surrounding Mrs Carter that she wasn't aware of, and Eloise felt she had a right to know if her new boss was somehow to blame for his wife's departure. She didn't want to work with someone who might have a temper, or other issues which had caused his wife to leave him. This was supposed to be a slower pace of life for her here, and she didn't need to get involved in any messy domestic situations. She'd had enough of her own to push through lately.

'Anne had brain cancer. Daniel was devastated after she died, obviously. They ran this clinic together. It was their baby, since they hadn't had any children. I don't know what he was like before he lost his wife, but I think he kind of withdrew into himself. He doesn't go out much and work seems to be his life.' Debbie clearly thought a lot of her colleague and seemed genuinely concerned for him.

'That's terrible.' Eloise had to admit, he hadn't given her the impression he was a sad, reclusive widower.

Then again, she'd been good at hiding her pain during the worst part of her life, not wanting her daughters to see it, or give her husband the satisfaction of knowing how much he'd hurt her. So she'd packed it all away inside and plastered on that brave face too—at least, until last night. Something had triggered the floodgates to open and she'd finally expressed all of her frustrations and fears which she'd bottled up all this time. Although it had been epically cringeworthy at the time, perhaps it would prove cathartic in some way, finally to have got it off her chest.

She supposed Daniel still had to deal with his grief and loss in his own way too.

'Yes, but he wouldn't like to think we're gossiping about him, I'm sure. I just thought it would be good for you to know, to try to avoid any misunderstandings.'

Eloise just about managed not to tell Debbie it was too late for that.

'Okay, I'll get your uniform sorted, and Debbie can give you the quick tour.' The receptionist disappeared out the back and left Eloise with the pretty vet.

'Obviously, this is the waiting room.' Debbie gestured round the bright, spacious room peppered with several chairs and posters of special dog-food and warnings about ticks.

Eloise followed her behind Reception, bypassing the small room which she knew was Daniel's office.

'We have a couple of examination rooms, our own theatre for minor surgeries and our pet hotel for overnight guests.' The whirlwind tour revealed the usual steel tables and medical equipment Eloise was familiar with.

If there had been a few more open doors or lights on last night, she might have seen inside and figured out for herself that Daniel was a vet, not a doctor. Though, perhaps she'd seen what she'd wanted to see. After everything she'd been through, the dam had been sure to burst at some point, and both she and Daniel had simply been unlucky that he'd been the one to witness it.

'I guess I'll pick up everything as I go along, though I'll probably have to get you to walk me through how you do things here.' Every practice had its own procedures, and she didn't want to overstep anywhere. She was probably going to have to work even harder to impress her new boss, now he knew what a disaster she was behind her immaculate CV.

'No problem. We're one big happy family here.' Debbie gave her a wide smile, reminding her why she was here. She liked these people, and the area. It was perfect for her new start, and she was going to have to get over last night's very vocal *faux pas* to make it work. She'd gone through a lot worse than oversharing with her new boss and survived. This was simply a blip.

'I'm looking forward to getting into the swing of things.' Maybe then she could relax.

'It won't take long. We're not exactly swamped. It's not like a big city vet. You'll probably spend more time chatting to the locals about the weather, or the rubbish the tourists have left behind, than treating their pets.'

'Suits me. I'm not cut out for long hours without a break. I'm hoping to wind down a bit at my age.'

Debbie turned and frowned at her. 'You're not old. Why does everyone over forty think they're past it these days?'

'Um, because we're made to feel that way.' If she hadn't already embarrassed herself with one work colleague by spilling the details of her personal life, she might've been tempted to do so now just to prove a point.

Neither Debbie nor Brooke were aware of the exact reasons she'd moved here, other than her daughters had moved out and she was on her own. She supposed 'why are you single again at your age?' wasn't on the list of approved interview questions these days. Though she was sure it wouldn't be long before they'd extracted the details, given that she'd already had the rundown on Daniel's circumstances.

One thing she'd neglected to factor in when moving to a small town was that gossip was the local source of entertainment. Boy, did she have some juicy tales with which to fuel the conversations around here!

'Well, you're not. You're shiny new around these parts and everyone will want to know all about you.'

Debbie confirmed her worst fears, making her shiver. It was bad enough that her boss knew how undesirable she was without the whole town knowing too, though they'd be able to see for themselves without having to strain their eyes too much. Her expanding waistline, hair in need of a wash and blow-dry and her hormonal acne breakouts would tell that story soon enough.

She made a note to unpack her hair straighteners and make-up bag as soon as possible. Today she'd had to make do with the powder compact, lipstick and eyeliner she carried in her bag for emergencies.

'First off, though, tea!' The receptionist handed her a uniform before directing her back towards the small staff room.

'We start every day with a cuppa.' Debbie flicked on the kettle, and Daniel appeared in the doorway the second it boiled.

'Who's turn was it today?' he asked.

'Yours,' the girls chorused, and he swore under his breath.

'Sorry, I forgot. I was out on a call last night and, well, I got distracted…'

He slid a glance at Eloise and she wondered what she was to blame for other than making them both uncomfortable.

'It's just as well we keep emergencies…' The receptionist opened the cupboard and reached in for a plastic tub, which when opened revealed a whole selection of yummy biscuits.

'We take turns buying, but Daniel has a habit of forgetting,' Debbie explained, giving him the side-eye.

He reached into his pocket, pulled out his

wallet and produced a five-pound note. 'Here, that should cover me for my next turn too.'

He set it on the counter before helping himself to some chocolate-covered digestives.

'Let me know when it's my turn to contribute,' Eloise insisted, accepting the cup of tea and biscuits offered to her. She had a feeling she was going to like working here, already being made to feel part of the family.

'We'll add you to the rota.' Debbie leaned against the kitchen counter, sipping casually, as though they had all the time in the world.

Eloise was used to a much more frantic pace of work, with a constant stream of pets and emergencies. This was what she needed—time for herself. She had to make herself a priority for once, and this place seemed perfect for that.

'How's the house?' Brooke asked.

'Good, although I've a lot of unpacking to do. I was lucky to get it fully furnished, but now I just have to find everything I brought with me.' She'd realised that this morning when she'd overslept and had had no idea where were her toiletries, kettle or any other morning essentials.

'We could all go over tonight and help you unpack,' Debbie suggested.

'I couldn't ask you to do that.'

'You didn't. Besides, we want to have a good nosy at the house, don't we, Debs? Daniel can put those muscles to work and do the heavy lifting and we could order a wee takeaway.' The receptionist was planning everyone's evening for them, and Eloise couldn't find a way to get out of it when she was being so kind.

'We don't want to steam-roll over Eloise when she's only just got here. She might have plans, or not feel up to having visitors just yet.'

There was something about Daniel's interference which got Eloise's back up, even though he was probably only trying to help. She couldn't help but think her revelation to him about her personal circumstances and health issues might have contributed in some way to his decision to pour cold water on Debbie's idea. Either that, or he was reluctant to spend any time with her outside of work again.

'I was just trying to help.' Debbie sniffed, her nose obviously out of joint at having had her idea shot down.

'I appreciate it. It would be lovely to have some help, and I haven't had time to do a food shop yet, so a takeaway sounds perfect. Only if Daniel wants to, of course.' She batted her eyelashes as she tossed the ball back into his court.

There was a flicker of reticence in his eyes before he responded. 'Sure. Dinner's on me.'

Eloise swallowed hard as she realised she'd just agreed to another night in her boss's company.

CHAPTER THREE

DESPITE THE FACT her new work colleagues were coming to help her sort out the house, Eloise found herself fussing around, trying to make it look as tidy and clean as possible—not an easy feat when everything was piled high in boxes. She had at least managed to locate the dishes and cutlery, unwrapping and washing them ready for use.

Her working day hadn't been too taxing, and she supposed they were breaking her in easy. Everyone had been very kind and patient with her as she got to grips with where everything was kept. She and Daniel hadn't interacted a whole lot unless it was work-related. He'd called for her assistance with a particularly difficult feline patient who'd objected to having its temperature taken, but between them they managed to coax it into co-operating. She'd taken blood samples, helped administer vaccinations and had even cut a pet rabbit's over-long front teeth, all whilst chatting away to the locals and getting to know their patients. Overall, it had been a fun, if tiring, day.

The doorbell rang and her stomach clenched, as though her date had just arrived, which was a silly thought. It was just nerves about opening up her new house to people she hardly knew. Of course, she'd also made sure to locate her favourite jeans, which hugged her ample butt, and her wrap-over black shirt with the red roses on it, which showed off her cleavage. Daniel had seen and heard her at her worst; it was only natural she should want to look nice. It didn't mean any more than that.

'Hi!' She opened the door to the trio, who all appeared to have travelled together.

'Well, give us the tour,' Brooke demanded the minute she set foot inside.

'Give her a minute,' Debbie insisted, following in behind.

Daniel was last in and simply gave her a nod in acknowledgement.

As he walked past she caught a whiff of his peppery aftershave, saw the crisp, ironed crease of his pristine pale-blue shirt and the shine on his shoes. It made her smile. Whilst the other members of the party had donned more appropriate scruffy jeans and ripped sweatshirts, it seemed Eloise and Daniel had both made more of an effort. At least she didn't appear to be the only one who wanted to make a good impression.

'Let me give you the guided tour first, then we can set to work putting the boxes in the right rooms at least.' After getting in so late last night, post-spilling her guts to Daniel, she'd been too physically and emotionally exhausted to do anything other than dump her belongings in the living room and fall into bed. Thank goodness she'd had the foresight when packing at least to label the cardboard boxes before chucking all of her worldly possessions into them.

'It's a good-sized room.' The receptionist spun round, arms wide like a child, to prove the point.

'Yes. I have to admit that's what sold it for me. The patio doors open out onto the decking with a lovely view of the loch.' She'd pictured herself sitting out there in the mornings with a coffee, enjoying the peace and quiet. It would be a world away from the busy main road where their family home had been. Although, that was how she'd been able to afford this place: a city centre two-up, two-down was in a very different price bracket. And there was something to be said for settling down young and having a mortgage paid out before the age of fifty.

Even after her husband had had his share, there had been just enough left for her to buy this place, and she had no intention of moving ever again. It had been traumatic to say the least, having to get rid of a lot of their things and closing the door on the place she'd called home for over two decades.

'Are you going to use the fireplace?' Debbie asked, inspecting the stone centrepiece of the room.

'I hadn't really thought about it. I have central heating, but it might be nice in the winter.' She could quite cosily curl up in here under a blanket with a book and a hot chocolate with no need for anything, or anyone else, in her life.

'You'll need to get someone qualified to make sure it's safe before you open that up.' Daniel was quick to issue the warning and she was touched that he was thinking of her safety—even if it was more likely that he thought she was daft enough accidentally to burn the place down because she hadn't checked to see if the chimney was blocked in any way first.

'Yes, I'll make sure to do that,' she said diplomatically, rather than start an argument over it.

'What do you need us to move first?' Daniel rolled up his sleeves, clearly ready to start, no doubt wanting to get this over with as soon as possible, since he'd been railroaded into it.

So much for the tour.

'I've already started unpacking some of the kitchen things—perhaps you could carry the heavier items in there for me, please.' The kitchen was her domain, and she'd acquired some expensive equipment over the years. Even though she wouldn't have a houseful of hungry teens, such as when her daughters used to bring their friends round, she might do some baking again if the mood took her. She'd prided herself on making good home-cooked food for her family when they were growing up. It had been sad when her daughters had moved out and she'd just been cooking for two.

By the time her marriage had ended, she hadn't had the same urge to make anything from scratch. Processed ready meals and takeaways probably hadn't helped her weight gain, either. However, she was hoping that out here, where access to supermarkets and takeaways was limited, she'd do more cooking. This new lifestyle out here seemed more conducive to exercise too. Hopefully, instead of simply sitting in front of the TV, she'd enjoy long country walks and maybe even some wild swimming.

Daniel certainly appeared to keep active. For a man of his age, he was clearly looking after himself. She'd seen the muscles flex as he'd rolled up his sleeves, and he certainly wasn't sporting the same rounded belly her ex had seemed to take great pride in at times. 'All bought and paid for,' Sam used to say, jiggling it.

Of course, her body wasn't the same as when they'd married either, but it hadn't seemed to matter to Sam that she'd birthed two children. He couldn't get past the physical changes in her during their thirty years together. Then menopause had arrived, determined to steal what was left of her femininity, and she hadn't felt very sexy.

Somewhere along the way, she supposed they'd both fallen out of love with one another. It had just taken her longer to realise it, accepting comfort and familiarity over passion, or even attraction—something which had become more apparent after the girls had moved out and it had been just the two of them left in the house. Perhaps Sam had been right to make the break and want something more for the rest of his life. Now Eloise just had to find her new place in the world without him.

'We'll just, er, unpack your books and ornaments for in here,' Debbie said when there was no further instruction.

'Sorry. I zoned out there for a moment.' Eloise blinked back into the room in time to see Daniel shifting with ease her heavy, expensive mixer, her other two colleagues staring at her.

'No problem. I'm sure it's been a long couple of days for you.' The receptionist put a reassuring hand on her arm before beginning to unwrap the more fragile items destined for the room.

'That's an understatement. I'm sure I'll be able to relax once I have all of my own things around me. If you could just unpack those onto the book shelves for now, I'll sort them out later. Thanks.'

'Aww, are these your daughters?' Debbie held up a framed photograph of her girls, which made her suddenly very emotional. It hit home that she was essentially starting this new part of her life without them, and that was very hard to do when she'd been there for them every day of their lives. For some reason this felt different from when they'd made the decision to leave home. She'd still been there, ready to welcome them back at a moment's notice, but now it was just her.

'Yeah: Dawn and Alison. They both live

abroad now. If you don't mind, I'm just going to take some of these boxes up to the bedroom.' She needed to get out of the room and compose herself before she made a fool of herself in front of Daniel again by blubbing and feeling sorry for herself.

Without waiting and having to explain why she was here without her family, Eloise grabbed the nearest boxes and hurried out of the room. Hopefully, some day it wouldn't hurt as much as it did right now to be here on her own.

'Where's Eloise?' Daniel asked, noticing her absence when he came back into the living room to collect his next assigned armful of his new nurse's belongings.

'She took some stuff upstairs to the bedroom,' Debbie informed him, continuing to line the book shelves with a selection of romcoms and thrillers. Eloise appeared to have an eclectic taste in reading habits.

It was good news for him that everyone was working away. He might have let himself be roped into this but that didn't mean he intended to make a night of it. It shouldn't take him long to shift a few boxes and, if the others wanted to stick around, he was more than happy to pay for a taxi to take them home. This was already more socialising than he usually did and he didn't want to give anyone the impression that this could be a regular thing—especially Eloise, when this was the second night they'd spent in one another's company. He'd already learned more about her personal life than he knew about those of the employees with whom he'd worked for years. He kept a distance from people for a reason.

After losing his mother when he'd been just thirteen, he'd gone into the care system. He barely remembered his father, who'd abandoned them when he'd been just four years old, so his whole adolescence had been spent moving from one foster home to another. He'd been too old for most people who wanted to adopt and create their own little family. No one wanted a troubled teen, so he'd learned to be self-sufficient, not getting too attached, because eventually he'd be separated from anyone he got close to.

It was only Anne who'd persuaded him to share his life with someone else. They'd met at a veterinary conference. Though she'd been older, they'd had the same focus on work, neither of them keen on starting a family. It had seemed logical to set up a practice together, as well as a new life.

They'd been happy living and working here, then Anne had been taken from him too. He'd learned his lesson and, since losing his wife, he'd lived a solitary existence outside of work. Last night Eloise had crashed into that existence, and now here he was, returning the favour. Hopefully after she was moved in he could get back to normality.

'Yeah, she seemed a little upset when we asked about her daughters,' his receptionist added, pointing out the framed photograph of Eloise and her girls.

Eloise was smiling, happier than he'd seen her so far, dwarfed by her tall, dark-haired clones. He could only imagine what it would be like to have a family of his own, but he did know how it felt when a family was no longer there. Okay, so her daughters hadn't passed away, but they weren't currently in her life, and she'd told him last night how sad she was. They had that in common.

Despite his wish to get out of here as soon as possible, he couldn't in good conscience leave her to wallow on her own. He was the only one who knew what she was going through, who understood to some extent how she felt. At the very least he should check on her.

'I'll go and see if she needs a hand,' he told

the others, resigned to the fact that he was probably the only person she could talk to about the things that were troubling her...whether he liked it or not.

Eloise took a moment to look at the contents of the boxes she knew were guaranteed to bring a tear to her eye. As well as the family photo albums she couldn't bear to part with, even though her husband was in most of the pics too, were the girls' toys and baby things.

She hoisted the box onto the un-made bed she'd fallen into last night, before she'd even had the chance to unpack the bedclothes, and peeked inside. There were the well-loved teddy bears, and the dolls who were now partially bald and covered in pen marks. There were the school reports and primary school paintings. All of them held memories of a better time, yet somehow it still seemed like only yesterday.

She supposed soon enough there would be grandchildren and other family get-togethers, and eventually she'd feel part of their lives again. Until then, she simply had to keep going on her own. They had their own lives to live now. Dawn lived with her husband in Australia, and Alison worked in Canada—too far away for a hug.

With a sigh, she closed the box back up. The best place for this was probably in the loft out of sight for now—at least until she could look at things without wanting to weep.

'Eloise?' Daniel knocked on the open door.

'Hey.' She did her best to compose herself again. As tempting as it was, falling into Daniel's arms in a sobbing mess wasn't going to do either of them any good. She was probably lucky he hadn't employed her on a trial basis or he'd be looking for ways to get rid of her, if she kept dragging him into her personal affairs. By all accounts he was a private man, and would likely prefer it if she kept her business to herself too.

'Debbie thought you seemed a bit upset. I just wanted to check that you were all right.' It was a kind gesture, though he was hovering in the doorway, apparently ready to make his escape at any moment. The girls had probably forced him to come up here and see how she was.

'I'm okay. Just missing my daughters, that's all.' She plastered on a smile and got up from the bed, lifting the box with her.

'It'll take a while to get used to. Not that you'll get used to being without them but you learn to adapt.' Although he was trying to comfort her, there was a sadness in the tone of his voice and a faraway look in those deep-brown eyes. He was thinking about his wife.

Eloise's heart went out to him. At least she could still talk to her daughters and see them every now and again, even if it was just on a video call. Daniel truly was on his own, and seemed unprepared to change that. She didn't want to end up the same, shut away completely from the rest of the world. Eloise simply wanted to come to peace with the fact this was her new life now, not become a recluse.

'Thanks. I'm just being silly and reminiscing over their childhood.'

As she shifted the weight of the box in her arms, a small teddy bear fell out at his feet. Daniel picked it up and smiled. It was a strangely sad expression which made her heart catch at the sight of it. 'It must be nice to have so many memories and mementos. I don't have anything like that. Mum died when I was thirteen and no one thought it was important to keep any of my childhood for me.'

'That's terrible. Don't you have anything?' She doubted the insight he was giving her into his background was a privilege he gave willingly to many, and it painted a bleak picture. Although both of her parents had died before she was married, she'd at least had a wonderful childhood and a lifetime of memories to cling onto.

'A few worn photographs, and my mother's sweet tooth.' This time the smile did reach his eyes, and it transformed his face completely, making him look like a little kid. It was the mischievous grin of someone who'd been found too often with his hand in the biscuit tin—something she could definitely relate to.

'I'm glad you have something to remember her by. It's important, even if it hurts to remember sometimes.'

Eloise tried to ignore the cute look, or the feelings she was beginning to have for her new boss, and reminded herself she hadn't even moved in to her new house. The last thing she needed was to jeopardise her job and her place here with an ill-advised, ill-timed and unwanted crush on someone she was going to work very closely with.

Apart from the fact he knew intimate details about her problems, she wasn't exactly in her first flush of youth. Daniel could probably have his pick of anyone around here, and someone still young enough to give him the family he seemed to have missed out on, even if he was ready to move on from the death of his wife. Which, given that it had been five years, and he didn't seem to leave the house unless it was an emergency call out, seemed as likely as him being attracted to her in return.

'Where do you want to put the rest of these?' He lifted another couple of the smaller boxes and followed her out onto the landing.

'I'm just going to put them in the loft for now. I'm not sure what it's like up there yet, but there's supposed to be a ladder for access at least.' She grabbed the pole propped up nearby which had a hook on the end, pulled on the steel ring attached to the trap door on the ceiling and let it fall back. The ladder immediately crashed down, sending her toppling out of the way and boxes flying everywhere.

'Easy,' Daniel said, as she stumbled straight into him.

For a moment they were locked in one another's arms, eye contact unwavering, breath held. It was as though time had somehow stood still and they were frozen in the moment. Eloise's mouth was dry as she gazed up into his heavy-lidded eyes, acutely aware of the strong hands which had caught her by the waist.

'I...er...let me take those up for you.' Daniel broke through the tense silence first, his voice hoarse, suggesting she hadn't imagined something happening between them.

'Be careful. As I said, I haven't been up there yet.'

She didn't argue with him. Ladders and dark places weren't her favourite things in the world, and a little personal space from him might help her to think clearly again, so her brain wouldn't be completely taken up with how long and pretty his dark eyelashes were, or how his lips looked so full and soft. Although, these new thoughts about a member of the opposite sex were a revelation that apparently she wasn't dead from the waist down—even if the discovery was at an inopportune time with the completely wrong person.

Maybe she wouldn't have to spend the rest of her days alone…if there was a middle-aged man somewhere out there desperate enough for company to settle for an overweight, menopausal divorcee.

With the first of the boxes tucked under his arm, Daniel climbed up the ladder, leaving Eloise unashamedly to ogle his backside: 'athletic', she would call it, not chunky or flat, and it filled his trousers nicely…

'Is there a light up here?' he called down after disappearing into the hole in her ceiling.

'They said there was… Try feeling along for a switch or a light pull.' She really ought to have paid more attention, but she'd been so excited by the forest view, the blue skies and the tranquil loch that things such as a light in the attic hadn't seemed important...until now.

Daniel's footsteps sounded above her, on what she hoped was floorboards. It would make storage so much easier if there was a fitted floor. She still had things such as luggage and her Christmas decorations to hide away up there. As she mused over the extra room she might have, there was a crashing sound, followed quickly by a very masculine, expletive-filled yell.

'Daniel? Are you okay?' she called up into the darkness.

'No. I think I've just fallen through your ceiling.' He sounded extremely calm, considering...

Eloise rushed into the bedroom, half-expecting to see Daniel lying there with debris all around, with a great big hole in the ceiling, but there was nothing. She checked in the spare room too but could see no sign of him there either.

'Daniel? I can't see you.'

'I'm definitely stuck here...' He sounded more ticked off than injured, so she hoped the damage both to him, or her ceiling, wasn't too great.

On impulse, she finally yanked open the doors to the built-in wardrobe in the spare room, only to be greeted with the sight of Daniel's legs hanging in the top of the closet. 'Oh, my goodness!' She hadn't meant to laugh, but really, it was like something out of a farce.

'I'm glad I'm amusing you, but apart from being stuck this is also kind of painful.' Though she couldn't see his face, Eloise could imagine the sardonic look on it.

'I'm coming,' she yelled up through the Daniel-shaped hole in her ceiling.

Despite her own anxiety about the ladder and the dark attic, she bounded up to go and help him. With the light still unlocated for now, she used the torch on her phone to guide her steps over to Daniel, who was wedged in between the joists.

'I'm so sorry,' she said, setting her phone down so she could use both hands to try and dislodge him from the plaster board.

'It's my own fault. I should have known better than to try and walk between the joists where there's nothing to support my weight.'

As Eloise hooked her hands under his arms and pulled, he pushed down until he finally came unstuck. He fell back on top of Eloise, his body crushing her.

'Daniel...' she croaked.

'Sorry.' He rolled off her, so they were lying side by side, her phone providing the only light.

Both were panting heavily, and for a moment she imagined that they could have been two lovers lying in post-coital bliss. A ridiculous notion, of course, but that was the sort of image this man conjured up in her fevered brain. Working together was going to prove a bigger challenge than simply pretending he didn't know about all the skeletons in her closet. At least she'd managed to keep this one to herself so far.

'Are you okay?' she asked, once she'd recovered from her physical exertion and her wandering thoughts.

He pulled up his shirt to reveal where he'd been battered and bruised during the escapade. 'It stings a little, but I'm sure I'll survive.'

Seeing the red marks on his skin, and the deep grazes he'd sustained while trying to help her, Eloise felt bad.

'I think we need to get you patched up. Everything else can wait.' She held out a hand and helped him to his feet, though he had to stoop under the eaves of the roof so he didn't knock himself out.

They gingerly came back down the ladder, and she led him into the bathroom.

'Sit here and I'll go and see if I can find a first-aid kit.' Eloise directed him to take a seat on the edge of the bath in the small bathroom.

'I'm sure I'll be fine. There's no need to put yourself to any trouble on my account.'

She ignored his protest, sure she'd seen the contents of her bathroom cabinet in a bag somewhere.

'Hey, Eloise, what was all the noise? Is everything all right?' Debbie asked when she walked back into the living room and began to rummage in the boxes again.

'Daniel had a bit of an accident,' she said, not prepared to go into details and give them any ammunition with which to tease him when she was sure he just wanted to forget about it.

'Is he okay?' Brooke piped up from behind the book she was currently reading instead of unpacking alongside Debbie. Not that Eloise could criticise, when they were all doing her a favour.

'A few scrapes. Nothing serious. I'm just looking for my first-aid kit... Ah, got it!' She grabbed her supplies and made a hasty exit before they could quiz her any further.

'Should we order dinner? I'm starving,' the receptionist called after her plaintively.

'Sure. My credit card is in my bag. Just use it to order whatever you want. My treat for helping.' It was the least she could do, and might keep them busy enough until she had Daniel sorted out and save a few of his blushes at least. She reckoned she owed him one when so far he'd kept her secrets for her.

He was still sitting where she'd left him, examining the grazes marring his side.

'The girls are ordering food. I reckoned that would keep them out of our way until I get you patched up.' Eloise gave her hands a quick wash then pulled out an antiseptic wipe to clean the badly grazed skin on his torso.

Daniel sucked in a breath through his teeth. 'I guess I should think myself lucky you didn't bring them up to film my mishap and find myself on one of those "funniest home video" shows.'

'Damn it. I could have made myself two hundred and fifty quid if I'd thought of that,' Eloise joked, ignoring the flash of his taut torso she was enjoying, and the feel of his warm skin beneath her fingers.

'Ow. Don't make me laugh. I think I bruised a couple of ribs on the way down.'

'Poor baby!' She pouted, before breaking out into a grin.

'I know. I'm being a brave soldier, you know.' Daniel gave her a brief glimpse of the jovial character she hadn't seen much since first meeting him, and she had to say she liked it. It was a sign that the man knew how to have fun, and wasn't as serious as he seemed on outward appearances.

'Just don't expect me to kiss it better,' she said, gently applying some antiseptic where the skin had been broken.

Only when she looked into his dark eyes, which were no longer twinkling with amusement, did she realise what she'd said. Now he was looking at her as though that was exactly what he wanted her to do and it was a jolt of lightning she hadn't been expecting, mostly because she didn't know what to do about it.

Of course she wasn't going to kiss him anywhere, but the fact that he might want her to wasn't something she'd anticipated. It was one thing being attracted to her new boss, but something else if he might actually feel it too. That was something neither of them could really afford to follow up. She stepped back and packed away her first-aid kit, quickly letting the moment dissipate.

'I'll owe you one.' His voice was even deeper than usual and Eloise was afraid to let her thoughts linger on what that 'one' could be.

'I think that makes us even,' she said, shutting down whatever this was happening in the confines of her small bathroom.

'The food's here!' their colleagues chorused from downstairs. She'd never been so relieved for food to take her away from an attractive man.

Daniel forced down several slices of pizza and the low-alcohol beer bought especially for him, regardless that he had no appetite. All he really wanted to do was get home to his safe space, his sanctuary, where he'd be content in his own company and wouldn't think about his new nurse kissing his bare skin...

'Would you like a taste?'

As three pairs of eyes turned to look at him across the living room, it occurred to him that Eloise had spoken and was now waiting for an answer.

'Excuse me?'

'I can see you staring at the Texas barbecue dip I'm hogging; would you like some?' She held up the little pot and he dipped the last bit of crust in it simply for appearances' sake.

'Thanks.'

It wouldn't do for anyone in this room to realise his head and thoughts had somehow been turned away from his late wife and onto the woman he'd just helped to move in. Although, Anne would've wanted him to move on—she'd always chided him for being so withdrawn from society—it felt like a betrayal even to be attracted to another woman. The two didn't even look alike—Anne a tall, slender blonde compared to the voluptuous woman with chestnut hair currently occupying his thoughts. He clearly didn't have a type, but there was something which he was drawn to. Of course, she was attractive but, more than that, he'd felt an instant connection to her from the moment she'd spilled all her personal problems out to him in his office.

Perhaps it was that recognition of her loneliness that had bonded them together. Though he hadn't admitted it to himself, life without Anne had been rather...quiet. He'd told himself he didn't need anyone else in his life. Anne had been a huge part of his every day and, now she was gone, no one could replace her. He wasn't prepared for anyone to fill that space, only for them to be taken from him again too. However, it was possible that he needed to expand his world beyond his practice.

Anne had been the one who'd thrown dinner parties for friends and colleagues, because they'd had no family to socialise with. It was she who'd accepted invitations to awards ceremonies, or booked the occasional weekend away. Daniel had never cared where he was, as long as he was with her. Once she'd gone, there'd seemed little point in pretending he wanted to be part of anything else. It wasn't long before the invitations had stopped coming, and he'd got used to being on his own again. As though he'd reverted back to that self-sufficient teenager no one had been interested in.

Tonight was the most sociable he'd been in five years, and it had served as a reminder why he didn't venture far from his own door. Making a fool of himself falling through the ceiling aside, he'd let his thoughts drift somewhere they shouldn't—to another woman. And not just any woman—his new nurse who, by her own admission, had problems of her own to work through.

Those few moments they'd shared alone, when she'd stumbled into his arms, and when she'd touched him in the bathroom, had wakened something in him. It wasn't just an attraction; he realised how much he'd missed that physical connection. He was sure he'd had moments when he'd brushed against other people in passing, and he shook a lot of hands in the context of his job, but there'd been something more to it when he and Eloise had touched. He'd wanted more, as though it had awakened a hunger in him that only she could satisfy. None of which had been the plan when he'd only agreed to move a few boxes for her.

'If it's okay, I'm going to head home.' Daniel broke through the quiet lull which had descended onto the room once they'd eaten their fill of carbs.

He'd organise a taxi for the others if they weren't ready to leave yet, but he didn't want to stick around in case any more little 'incidents' occurred between Eloise and him. Hopefully, if they kept their relationship strictly on work premises, he wouldn't misinterpret any close contact for anything likely to jeopardise his current peace of mind.

'Me too. Sorry, Eloise, I'm shattered.' Thankfully Debbie also got to her feet, with a yawn, so he didn't look as if he was being the party pooper.

'Maybe we can pick this up at the weekend?'

Brooke suggested, though Daniel hoped she was only being polite. The last thing he wanted to do was spend the weekend dodging whatever this was building between Eloise and him.

'No, you've all done plenty. Thank you so much.' She saw them to the door and, though Daniel felt guilty about the empty pizza boxes and cans they'd left behind, he was glad to leave. Glad to go back to his quiet, empty home where he didn't have to worry about anyone else but himself.

Daniel opened the car for the other two to get in, social etiquette requiring he at least showed his appreciation to his host for dinner before he scarpered.

'Thanks for dinner. My turn next time.' To his horror, he found himself offering an invitation to do this again. Worse, he leaned in and kissed her on the cheek, as though his body had been taken over and he had no control of his actions.

He walked back to the car, eyes wide, heart pounding, a small part of him looking forward to doing it all again.

CHAPTER FOUR

'HELLO.'

'Lovely day, isn't it?' Eloise gave a nod in passing to a couple walking hand in hand past the lake in the opposite direction, taking in the view.

The one thing she hadn't counted on when choosing her slice of solitude to live on was how many other people came to visit. For the most part it didn't interfere too much with her day-to-day living, but there was the odd inconsiderate tourist who left their litter at the side of the road, or the bikers who used it as a race track.

At least she lived on the other side of the road from the loch so it wasn't as though she had bus-loads of day-trippers parked in her drive-way. It was still a relatively quiet spot compared to where she used to live. Here, she could walk across the road without fear of being run over by an articulated lorry, and breathe in fresh air that wasn't polluted with diesel fumes. There were designated camping areas and laybys further on round the loch which people used.

People liked to come and enjoy an uninterrupted view of the sky without the light pollution of the city, which she had to admit was spectacular. She couldn't be selfish about sharing this place when she was just a blow-in from Glasgow herself. It was a good place to go for long walks to clear the head, especially on her day off after a week of awkward tension between her and Daniel.

The night everyone had helped her move in had been overwhelming in ways she could never have dreamed of. Apart from them being the most people with whom she'd spent time in company since her marriage had split, there had been those intimate moments alone with Daniel—not that they'd done anything other than exchange a couple of intense looks. Okay, so she might have taken more than a passing interest in his body when he'd lifted his shirt for her to tend to his injuries after his mishap, but that was only natural, wasn't it? He was a good-looking man and she'd been curious. And she had not been disappointed…

Eloise gave herself a mental shake, trying to dislodge that particular memory and the feel of his hard body beneath her fingers. Easier said than done when he'd ended the night kissing her on the doorstep. It might've been nothing more than a thankful peck on the cheek for dinner, but the touch of his lips on her skin had been branded there ever since.

She raised her hand and traced the very spot, as she did absent-mindedly when she recalled the event. She thought it had surprised both of them, it had been so out of the blue, and certainly hadn't been mentioned since, along with the offer of dinner. An invitation which she'd lain awake at night veering between wanting to accept, or run away from, should it ever come to fruition. In the end she needn't have worried. It had become clear by the next morning that nothing could've been further from Daniel's mind than spending any more time with her.

He'd been careful since not even to end up alone in the break room with her. That didn't mean he wasn't professional and courteous when they were working together, but somewhere along the way a line had been drawn between them. It wasn't a bad thing, when the feelings she'd begun to have towards a man she hardly knew were confusing and making her new life difficult. This was not what she wanted, or what she'd come here for.

'Should've known it was too good to last.'

The couple who'd passed her earlier were now rushing back the way they'd come, pulling the hoods of their rain coats over their heads as they ran towards their car.

Eloise had been so lost in her own thoughts she hadn't noticed the rain, but now she could see it dapple the water in the loch, hear it pitter-patter through the trees, feel it soak her skin and smell that fresh, earthy aroma it brought with it. Instead of rushing away from it, she embraced the downpour as a baptism of her new life here. It was a reminder that she was still alive, even if at times it had felt as though she'd died inside and she'd just kept going for the girls' sake. Slowly, she was beginning to live again.

She was sure this awkwardness around Daniel was simply part of the process of coming back to life. A realisation that she was still a woman, with feelings and needs which had lain dormant for a while due to everything going on in her chaotic life prior to moving. Things would settle down, and she was sure whatever her hormones made her think about her new boss would pass too. For now, she should concentrate on her, and getting her new house into some kind of order.

As Eloise made her way home, the beautiful purple and green hues of the landscape turned a muted grey. A heavy fog began to descend, cloaking her pretty view. She could just about see the road and the glow of car fog-lights ahead.

Suddenly, a deafening thud filled the air, quickly followed by the screech of brakes and an awful canine yelp. Eloise rushed to the side of the road just in time to see the car speed off again into the gloom, leaving the dog it had hit lying in the middle of the road. Making sure there were no other cars coming, she ran over to check on the poor pooch. Even though it was whimpering and in obvious pain, it was trying to lick her face.

'Oh, you're a sweetie, aren't you?' It was covered in dirt and blood, its fur matted and body emaciated, and it was hard to tell what breed it was, but it needed help regardless.

She scooped the dog into her arms, which for the size of it wasn't as heavy as it probably should've been. There was no collar or tags on its neck, and she doubted if they'd find a microchip. The poor thing looked as though it had been living rough for quite a while.

Although it was Sunday, the clinic closed and the staff enjoying their day off, she knew there was one man who'd still be on site. She reckoned Daniel would forgive her for crashing in on him, since this was an emergency, and he was always on call when it came to work.

'Don't worry, we'll get you sorted.' After laying the dog on the back seat of her car, she gave him a gentle stroke and was rewarded with a lick of her hand. Her heart broke for him, and at the same time rage was building up inside her that he'd been left in such a state. Now it was down to Daniel and her to make a difference to him and show that not all humans were capable of such cruelty.

Daniel turned off the shower, certain he heard a noise. He waited, suds still in his hair, listening until he heard it again: a desperate, rapid thumping on his front door. It wasn't unheard of for worried pet owners to turn up at his door out of hours but he couldn't very well greet them like this. He quickly rinsed off and grabbed a towel.

'Daniel? It's Eloise.' She sounded panicked.

After the strained atmosphere between them this week, he knew she wouldn't have come here unless something was seriously wrong. He wrapped the towel around his waist and padded, wet and barefoot, to the front door. The last thing he expected was to see her carrying a bleeding dog in her arms.

'He was hit by a car.' The anguish in her voice was reflected in the worry lines across her forehead.

'Bring him through to the surgery. I'll run and put some clothes on.' He let her into the house and unlocked the adjoining door into the clinic.

As he left, he heard her whispering soothing assurances to the injured animal. She was a great addition to the team, good with animals and their owners. It was only the vet who was having issues with her appointment.

He didn't know what on earth had come over him the other night when he'd kissed her on the cheek and casually thrown out a dinner invitation. It was almost as if his body had been possessed by someone who did that sort of thing all the time—not a grieving widower who'd been hiding away from the world for five years.

Thankfully, neither incident had been mentioned since. They'd both seemingly been resigned to things they would never speak of again, along with what had happened that first night they'd met.

However, it didn't mean he hadn't thought of that doorstep goodbye, and what might've happened in other circumstances—if he wasn't still grieving, so afraid of getting close to someone else. It might be nice to have dinner out with Eloise, like a normal man. Even if there was a possibility she'd be receptive to the idea when she'd obviously been scarred by her past relationship too. The fact that she hadn't even mentioned the matter in passing suggested that she thought it better forgotten too. Though, for a brief moment when he'd seen her on his doorstep, he'd thought it might be a social call, and the thought hadn't been as frightening as he'd have imagined.

'He's not microchipped. I think he's a stray,' Eloise told him when he came into Theatre.

He'd had to dress quickly and his clothes were still clinging to his wet skin. Not ideal conditions to work in, but this was clearly an emergency.

'We'll need to X-ray him and probably open him up to fix the fracture. I can already see the bone sticking out through the injury sight so I'm going to need to set that.' An open fracture like that was a high risk for infection and could cause complications if not closed and reset properly.

'Even if he's a stray?' It was clear Eloise was already attached to the dog, and her likely concerns about costs were understandable.

'Even if he ends up in the dog home, I'll still

do whatever it takes to have him back on his paws.' Daniel gave her a smile to reassure her that this was more than a business to him. He would never turn away an injured animal. It was the one area of his life over which he had any control, where he could make a difference without getting too attached. Although the animals sometimes held a piece of his heart, the best part of his day was seeing them go home happy and healthy. Though he didn't relish the idea of sending a dog to be rehomed, it had a better chance of being adopted if it had been seen and treated by the vet first, without passing on those costs.

They both donned their protective green scrubs. The X-rays showed a fractured femur to the front right leg, and Daniel was keen to operate straight away. Eloise shaved the area which was going to require surgery so Daniel could better see what he was doing.

'They always look so vulnerable, lying there,' Eloise remarked as she monitored the anaesthesia, preparing for surgery. Sometimes anaesthesia was the most dangerous part, depending on the dog's age and health.

Daniel couldn't argue. Head back, tongue lolling out of the side of its mouth, this little dog was completely at their mercy. At least they weren't going to let him down. By the look of it, the dog hadn't been cared for properly in a long time, and now it had been left for dead. It was Daniel's job to make sure that didn't happen.

'Hopefully, he'll be up and running around soon.' Daniel made the first incision and set to work trying to locate the piece of bone which needed to be put back in place.

'And then what? The dog's home?' Eloise's tone was accusatory, but if he kept every stray animal that came through the doors he could be a local tourist attraction.

'Well, we can put some posters up—see if anyone's missing him or willing to take him in. We'll cross that bridge when we come to it. For now, I just want to make sure our little friend recovers from his trauma.'

'He'll have to stay in for observation for a while, won't he?'

'I expect so.'

'Good. It's about time someone took care of him.' Eloise stroked his paw and proved again what an asset she was to the practice.

Although she was very capable at assisting him here in surgery, it was important that she was empathetic with the pet owners who needed their help. Everyone who came in through the door wanted to be sure that their well-loved fur babies were in good hands, that they were being treated by people who cared for them and thought of them beyond the bill at the end of the treatment.

Eloise was that special kind of person with room in her heart for everyone—human and animal. He was already enjoying working with her. She brought a new element to the place, a bridge between the other staff and him, as well as the patients. He was able to relate to her more than he had to anyone else in five years, even if that was bringing its own challenges.

'Can you hold that in place for me?' he asked Eloise as he prepared to drill into the two bits of bone, reconnecting them with the aid of some metal screws.

'Of course.' With a steady pair of hands, she held the fracture together until he'd finished pinning, then he was able to close up the site and wrap a bandage around the area.

'I'll keep an eye on him through the night just to make sure there's no infection.' There was always a risk post-surgery and, like a lot of the animals which were kept overnight, this dog would have to be monitored closely. High temperature or vomiting would require imme-diate treatment, so he kept a close watch on any overnight boarders. It wasn't as though he had anything else to do with his time, and it was a routine he and Anne had got used to along the way. It was as though these animals which had passed through had been their own little family, if only for a short while.

'Thanks,' Eloise said absentmindedly, as though he'd personally offered to do her a favour. She'd already bonded with their patient; she was a natural nurturer, which he was sure made her a great mum to her daughters. It was a shame for her that they didn't currently seem to be in her life, and he could only imagine the pain it caused her. They were both alone, but knowing she had family out there that she couldn't be with must hurt too.

'OK, we'll try and bring him round again. Careful, in case he's a bit disoriented.' Sometimes animals lashed out when the anaesthetic wore off, and stray dogs were the most unpredictable. The last thing he wanted was for Eloise to get hurt when she'd likely saved this pooch from dying a horrible death in the middle of the road.

'I think the only danger is that he might lick me to death.' Even as they carried him to one of the crates to settle him in bed for the night, he was nuzzling her. Clearly the infatuation was a two-way deal. Perhaps Eloise was going to be the one who'd end up with a house full of waifs and strays when she had so much love to give.

'He'll probably sleep for most of the night but I'll check in on him periodically to make sure he's all right,' he assured her when it became obvious she didn't want to leave the dog on his own.

Eloise made sure there was water for him and tucked a blanket around him. She probably would have read him a bedtime story if left to her own devices too.

'I think he needs a name.'

'I'm not sure that's a good idea. You don't want to get too attached, Eloise.' Regardless that it was already a lost cause.

'But it doesn't seem right, leaving him here in the dark and not even giving him a name.'

Daniel didn't know what difference it would make but if it kept Eloise happy, and more importantly got her to leave, he was happy to go along with it.

'Dan's a good name.'

She gave him a scathing look. 'No human names; it's weird. And nothing boring like Rex, or Prince.'

'Lucky?'

She gave an exasperated sigh.

'No, hear me out. Not only did he have a

lucky escape, but he was lucky you were the one to find him and bring him here.' Regardless of his insistence that neither of them should get too attached, Daniel had already put some thought into the idea too.

'Hmm, I suppose so. What do you think, Lucky? Do you like that?' She put her hand into the cage to give him one last stroke and the dog licked her in approval.

'Lucky it is, then. At least until we find him a permanent home somewhere else.'

The look she gave him was of utter betrayal on his part and he knew that Lucky was going to stick around for some time to come.

CHAPTER FIVE

'MORNING.' ELOISE BREEZED into the clinic and straight in to visit Lucky, as she had done every morning since his arrival.

Daniel no longer seemed surprised to see her this early, always dressed and ready to greet her, unlike the night when she'd first brought the dog to his door. The sight of him clad only with a towel around his waist, body wet, was an image not easily forgotten.

'Do you want some breakfast?' he called through from the annex. It had become almost commonplace now for her to be in his private part of the building before work. He usually had the kettle on for her arrival, and Lucky had somehow managed to help them bypass the awkwardness of being alone. They had something else to focus their attention on.

'I don't want to put you to any trouble.' She insisted every morning that she didn't want to intrude, she was only here to check on their patient, but as usual Daniel dismissed her protest.

'Tea's ready and I've got some toast on anyway. You can bring the mutt in with you, if you want…' His invitation would have been more of a surprise if she hadn't already spotted some dog toys lying around, evidence that he'd been keeping Lucky company outside of his usual working hours. It seemed she wasn't the only one with a soft spot for the dog.

'He's looking good this morning,' she commented as Lucky ran as fast as his bandaged leg would let him, straight from the surgery onto the sofa in the living room. She suspected he'd come to think of the place as his own, right in front of the television.

He'd also had a makeover of some kind. His coat was no longer matted with dirt and blood and was now a shiny golden mane, making him look cared for. Apart from the shaved patches where they'd operated on him, and the bandage on his leg, no one would know the trauma he'd been through.

'I…er…gave him a quick shower. Didn't want him stinking the place out.' Daniel dodged eye contact as he set to work buttering the mountain of toast on the breakfast bar in front of him where they'd taken to having their first cuppa in the morning—the one before the others came to work which no one else knew about.

Eloise grinned. Bathing the dog was something he could easily have tasked one of them to do during working hours. She suspected he was simply enjoying the company, as was she.

'I think he's put on a bit of weight too. He doesn't look as skinny as when he first came in.' Eloise was glad to see it. Ribs shouldn't be visible on a dog this size; it was a clear indication of malnutrition. Goodness knew how long the poor thing had been wandering around out by the loch, with very little to live on. Unlike the city, there wasn't the abundance of rubbish or leftover takeaways for him to rummage in for sustenance.

'That'll be down to the chicken breast you cook for him every day, on top of the meals he's getting.' Daniel pushed the cup of tea and plate of buttered toast towards her, and she sat on one of the high stools at the counter.

'And those have nothing to do with it, I suppose?' Eloise nodded towards the open bag of dog treats sitting on the kitchen worktop.

'Guilty as charged.' Daniel's blush was endearing.

'I suppose he'll be moving on soon.' Breaking off a piece of toast to feed to Lucky, who was patiently waiting at her feet, she broached the subject she'd been dreading.

'I'm afraid so. He can't take up a bed in the clinic indefinitely, but no one has come forward to claim him.'

It wasn't surprising, really, that whoever owned him hadn't admitted to the cruelty he'd obviously suffered, but it did mean that he'd have to be sent to the dog's home, with no guarantee that he'd be adopted. She didn't want to contemplate the alternative.

'You could keep him,' she suggested, since he appeared to have a home here anyway. Daniel seemed to enjoy having him around too.

He shook his head. 'There's a reason I never had a pet here. It wouldn't be fair to leave it alone all day. I get a lot of call outs. What about you? Couldn't you give him a home?'

'I'd love to, but I've got work too. You're right, it wouldn't be fair to keep him locked up all day.' Although, she supposed it wasn't going to be much different for him if he went to the dog's home.

'I guess I have no choice but to contact the dog warden to come and pick him up.' Daniel's heavy sigh, along with the half-eaten toast he pushed to one side, suggested he wasn't looking forward to that happening any more than she was.

'It's a shame when he seems to be thriving here. He's such a lovely guy.' Eloise stroked his soft fur, knowing he'd be great for cuddles when he wasn't so tender. It would be nice to share a sofa with him at night, like having a great big teddy bear to keep her warm. Having a dog in the house might make the place seem a lot less empty, and she wouldn't be talking to the walls the way she was now.

Except there was the problem of what to do with him during the day. It had been the same when the girls were little and they'd begged to have a puppy. She just hadn't had the time to spend at home; she'd always been working. There'd been bills to be paid, after all.

'I think we had a dog when I was little. I don't remember a whole lot, but I think he used to sleep in bed with me.' A half-smile crossed over Daniel's lips as the memory sprang to mind.

'What happened to him?'

'I'm not sure. Maybe my dad took him when he left. I've no one to ask. For all I know, he's nothing more than a figment of my imagination. I would've done anything to have a pet. Probably for that feeling of being loved, and having someone in my life. We weren't allowed any in the foster homes.' It was another sad glimpse at the lonely life he'd had as a teen, apparently with no family or friends to keep him company.

Eloise supposed it explained a lot about the way he interacted with people now. She could see it would be difficult for him at times when conversation with pet owners strayed beyond the realms of animal care. He didn't like to give a lot away about himself, and she knew even her being here in his home was likely a great test of his strength. He'd only agreed to it so that Lucky would benefit from having both of them to look after him.

'It's a wonder you don't have a house full of them now,' she mused. There was plenty of space, and opportunity, for him to have as many pets as he could ever want. She had to admit it was tempting for her to fill the house with replacements in her affections now that she didn't have her family around her to fuss over.

'Why do you think we made it our first rule when Anne and I set up the clinic not to literally bring our work home with us?' He grinned, and she could see he'd been trying hard to keep that particular impulse at bay for a long time too.

'What if…we both take him on?' Eloise couldn't believe she was suggesting this when, until Lucky came on the scene, they'd been try-

ing to keep their relationship strictly professional. However, she couldn't bear to think of
their canine companion going back into a world
where he wouldn't have special treats or evenings in front of the telly.

Worse, she wouldn't have anything to look
forward to in the mornings. She was referring
to seeing Lucky, not having breakfast with Daniel, obviously.

'How's that going to work?' It wasn't an
outright 'no', at least. Though neither of them
clearly wanted to commit full-time to the responsibility of having a dog, this compromise
might be a less intimidating prospect.

'Well, he could come to work with us. I'm
sure he wouldn't be any bother. We can take
turns walking him on our down time. One of
us could take week nights and the other could
take weekends,' she suggested with a shrug. It
was all the same to her when she didn't have
anything of a social life anyway.

'Like shared custody?'

'I guess so. At least until we decide otherwise. Circumstances might change, or one of
us might decide we're ready to be a full-term
pet owner further down the line.' She could see
that full-time owner being her, once she was
settled into her house properly, and having a

dog might make it feel even more like a home. It was just too soon in her chaotic life to be fair to Lucky when she still had a lot to sort out in her head, as well as her house.

Daniel studied the dog, who was looking at him adoringly, as though deciding whether or not he was worth the risk. It was no wonder he was still single if it took him this long to ponder whether to let a dog into his life on a part-time basis, never mind another partner. Not that Eloise could say anything when she was in exactly the same predicament. A dog wouldn't tire of her, or decide she wasn't worth loving any more. As long as she kept feeding it, at least.

'I suppose we could give him a trial, and if it doesn't work out...' Daniel didn't have to say any more. They both knew what the alternative was, and the thought of abandoning Lucky again sent a chill up her spine. After all, she knew how it felt to be rejected, found wanting and left on the scrap heap. If she could help a creature feel loved again, it would give her a sense of achievement. Even if she wasn't likely to experience that feeling for herself again.

'Best behaviour, buddy,' she warned Lucky with a wagging finger. Then felt guilty when he looked at her with those big, sad eyes. She gave him a cuddle so he knew she wasn't mad at him, though he'd never comprehend just how much she and Daniel were putting on the line to give him a home.

For a man she worried was already disrupting the new life she'd planned for herself here, she'd just made an arrangement which would bring them closer than ever. Hopefully, she could forget those feelings she'd been having for her boss in favour of caring for this little dog who so desperately needed a home.

Eloise wondered if she did just need something to focus her attention on, and she'd latched onto Daniel first. She'd spent her whole life looking after her family; it was only natural there would be a void in her life now she was living on her own. Hopefully, Lucky would fill that hole in her life, now her children were off exploring the world themselves. Then perhaps she'd get over this crush on her new boss and she could find the peace she was looking for.

'So, what, you're Lucky's parents now?' Debbie was clearly amused by the information, and no wonder when Daniel had spent years denying that he needed the company any time she'd tried to foist an abandoned pup or kitten onto him as though he was some sort of sad case desperately in need of a friend.

'Sort of. We've agreed to take care of him between us, that's all.' He tried to downplay it, even though it was the biggest commitment he'd taken on since he'd lost Anne.

It wasn't just because the stray needed a place to call home; goodness knew his heart strings had been tugged by many similar sob stories over the years and he'd managed to remain resolute. He didn't think it was even because he was now used to having a TV buddy in the evenings to share snacks with and watch football. No, a big deciding factor was Eloise. He could see how much the dog meant to her, and how torn she was about potentially having to say goodbye.

After everything she'd been through, he reckoned she could do with something nice happening to her for a change. Yes, initially it was going to mean being in each other's lives more than he'd been prepared for, but he hoped ultimately that Lucky would prove a distraction for both of them from the loneliness which was obviously drawing them together.

A pet was just something else for him to love and lose. He'd seen the devastation the death of his patients caused their owners. It could be like losing part of the family. That was the primary reason he hadn't been able to bring himself even to commit to a four-legged companion in the wake of Anne's death. His hope was that Eloise would eventually take over sole owner- ship once she was ready. She was the one who wasn't used to being alone, not him.

'It'll do you good to open up and share your life again,' Debbie said, casually sorting through her files on the reception desk, but Daniel cold hear the implication there.

'It's just a dog— a stray. For all we know, the owner will turn up next week looking for him.' He purposely focused on Lucky, rather than the fact she was alluding to Eloise, not wanting to fuel any workplace gossip.

'Uh-huh. And if they don't?'

'Then Eloise and I will continue to look after the dog the way we have been doing. It's no big deal. We both have a lot of spare time on our hands and it seemed logical to offer assis- tance, rather than see him go to a rescue cen- tre.' Sometimes he wished their little country practice had a bigger clientele so he didn't have to stand around discussing his personal life in between patients.

'Where is he now? I haven't seen him around this morning.'

'Eloise took him out for a walk whilst it's quiet. She'll be back soon, once she's settled him back in the house.' Despite Lucky's injury, it was necessary to take him out for restricted, slow walks to help him recover. They'd agreed to take turns, but Daniel would likely have the heavier workload during the day. At least it meant in any down time they had would most likely be spent apart and he could stop worrying about being in close contact with her all day, every day.

'She has a key to your house?' Debbie's eyes couldn't have been any wider than if he'd told her they'd eloped to Las Vegas over the weekend and got married.

'For the dog,' he reiterated with a scowl.

'For the dog,' she repeated with an annoying grin.

Daniel grabbed up the file for his next patient.

'Pinky Patterson,' he called to the one elderly lady sitting in the waiting room, with a shivering chihuahua in her handbag, ignoring Debbie's sniggering behind him.

He didn't mention Debbie's comments to Eloise when she returned. It would only annoy her. This arrangement was between them, nobody else's business, and he would've told his colleague that if he hadn't thought it would pique her interest in their deal with the dog even more. It was better just to let the matter drop than make a bigger fuss.

'Lucky's doing really well. He was obviously house trained wherever he started out, and he's walking to heel. Now we just have to get him to stop him trying to jump on people.' Eloise was flicking through the photos she'd taken of him on the short walk, like a proud parent.

'He might need some obedience classes once he's healed.' Daniel stopped short of volunteering to take him personally. That would be a step too far into commitment.

'Aww, it's not his fault. He's just desperate to be loved. It's his version of a hug.'

There was no doubt he was a loving dog, but not everyone would appreciate his attention at full force.

'Well, we can't run the risk of him knocking anyone over in his enthusiasm to say hello. I'm sure we have some details of local classes somewhere.' Daniel began rifling through the contents of the reception desk, Brooke being on her lunch break.

'Help me. Someone please help.' A young woman suddenly burst in through the surgery doors carrying a clearly distressed ginger cat in her arms, a trail of blood dripping onto the floor in their wake.

'Come on through.' Daniel opened the door to let her straight into the operating theatre, so he could have a good look at what was going on, with Eloise following behind.

'What happened?' she asked the woman gently, taking the cat from her arms to put him on the examination table.

'It was a dog, off the lead; it attacked him in the front garden. Marmalade was just lying enjoying the sun, and the next thing this devil dog was shaking him like a rag doll in its mouth. I had to fight him off myself until the owner eventually turned up and took him home. Not even a word of apology.' The woman was shaking, her arms covered in scrapes and grazes, clearly in shock.

'Well, he's in the best hands now. Why don't I get you settled with a nice cup of sweet tea and Daniel will check him over?' Eloise took her by the arm and led the woman out of the room. He knew she'd come back to assist him once she'd calmed down Mrs Gillies, as much a help to the concerned pet owners as she was to the animals, and to him.

The injured cat was uncharacteristically subdued and, though it made it easier for him to do an examination on his own, it was a clear sign that there was something seriously wrong. Cats in general weren't known for co-operating, and he'd suffered many a deep scratch in the line of duty. He managed to clean away some of the blood one-handed, whilst searching for the wound site. Unfortunately, he discovered several, deep and extensive, meaning there could be muscle or nerve damage as well as the possibility of infection.

'I hope you don't mind, but I've tucked her up in your office for now with a blanket and a cup of tea. I've asked Brooke to keep an eye on her until we're done here.' Eloise washed her hands and donned a plastic apron before joining him, holding their patient in place so he could do a thorough examination.

'That's great. Thank you. I think we can suture these more superficial wounds, but I'm worried there's some internal damage. We might need to open him up.' It was risky for an animal this age to be put under anaesthetic and he would have to get Mrs Gillies' consent before he did that.

'Shall I give him some pain meds?' Eloise was already preparing with the vial and needle, always thinking ahead.

'Yes, please.' He let her do that first, then set

to the task of closing up some of the puncture wounds caused by the dog bites.

Even when the cat was sedated, Eloise was stroking it, murmuring words of comfort. She worked differently from Anne and the veterinary nurses he'd employed in the past. This was obviously more than a job to her: she cared. Not that this was a profession a person could be in if they didn't have that empathy with the animals they treated, but Eloise took it to a different level, treating every pet with the same kindness and respect that was normally reserved for human patients.

He imagined the problem with having a heart that big was how painful it was when it was broken. She didn't deserve what had happened to her, and he hoped she found some peace here. As long as it didn't interfere with his.

'Mrs Gillies should probably report the incident to the police. Once we're finished here, I'll have a chat with her, make sure she's okay to do that.' Eloise was noticeably still worried about the owner, as well as her cat.

'Good idea. If a dog capable of that sort of attack is on the loose, there's always a chance it could hurt something, or someone, else.' Although the chances of finding the dog responsible or its owner were slim, it would still be advisable to report the incident in case it happened again.

'This sort of thing happened all the time in the city. I don't know why people take on dogs if they're not prepared to put the hard work in to train and look after them properly.' Eloise didn't talk much about her life in Glasgow, at least not since that first night when she'd mistaken him for a GP. It made Daniel curious about why she'd given that life up to move here on her own.

For him, it had been a compromise. Anne had wanted to open a practice, but he hadn't wanted to do so in a well-populated area. Although he'd grown up in and around Ayr town centre, he much preferred the quiet country life: less people, traffic and noise, as well as the space he needed for himself.

Growing up in care had been claustrophobic at times. Sharing rooms with others had made it difficult to have any personal space, regardless that he still felt emotionally isolated from those around him. A constant stream of house mates—different faces, each with their own issues and demons—hadn't provided him with any sense of stability or belonging. Opening up, showing any vulnerability, would only have made him prey for those who sought to exploit anyone who showed weakness. He'd seen it for himself: those who'd been abused in their own lives going on to repeat the pattern and become the abusers themselves, taking advantage of anyone they deemed inferior, using fists and words to pummel their victims into submission.

So he'd kept himself to himself. He'd put his head down and concentrated on his studies so he could break free of the system and make a life for himself. Except it had been difficult ever to escape that protective shell he'd wrapped around himself. Anne had been the only one to coax him out of it every now and then to join the real world. Although, somehow, Eloise had already managed to get him to agree to take on a pet...

'It must be a big change to come here. In general, I mean. What made you decide on this place?' He understood that need for change, to start again, but it didn't explain why she'd specifically come to this town. For him, it wasn't too far from the place he'd known his entire life, yet offered him the tranquillity he craved. Eloise was used to the bustling city, a house full of family, and this didn't seem the obvious place to start over. If anything, she would feel the loneliness more. He should know.

A soft smile lit up her face. 'I used to come

here with my parents when I was little. We had some great camping holidays at Loch Bruce.'

'Ah, the old rose-tinted spectacles...' It was easy to look back and think only of the good times. He was probably guilty of doing that where his marriage to Anne was concerned, skipping over the difficult parts to hold onto the good stuff, lest those memories of lost loved ones be tainted in any way.

'Perhaps, but I needed something positive to cling onto. There were too many bad memories for me in the city. I tried to carry on, living in the same area, doing the same job, but I was unhappy. This is where I remember being happiest.'

Daniel met her sad eyes, recognising that longing to go back, but knowing deep down it could never happen. 'I hope you find the contentment you're looking for.'

'So far, so good. I think Lucky will help keep me from wallowing too much in my own misery.' At least now there was a ghost of a smile on her face, and Daniel knew he'd made the right decision concerning the dog, regardless that he'd had second thoughts from time to time.

'He's certainly a distraction.' Daniel chuckled. His daily schedule had changed dramatically simply trying to keep him fed, entertained and keep the tumbleweeds of dog hair at bay.

'If it's okay, I'll collect him and his things when we're done here.' It was clear she was looking forward to having him to herself over the weekend. Their arrangement was very much like a divorced couple sharing custody of a child, only without any bad feeling or history.

'Of course.' Though Daniel had a feeling it was going to be a quiet weekend for him without his new charge around the house.

CHAPTER SIX

ONCE THEY'D FINISHED the surgery on Marmalade, they informed Mrs Gillies they'd be keeping him in overnight for observation. Eloise made sure she had someone to come and collect her after the shock of the attack, then they were able to lock up for the night.

'We'll see you two tomorrow,' Brooke said, looking pointedly at Eloise and Daniel.

Eloise felt herself blush, even though she'd done nothing wrong, and saw the dark look on Daniel's face at the suggestion there was anything going on between them. Thankfully Debbie appeared, waving a leaflet in Daniel's face to break the tension in the air.

'Don't forget the fete at the village hall tomorrow afternoon, either.'

'I haven't said for definite I'm going. I have a clinic to run.' Daniel snatched the piece of paper from her hand.

'What's this?' Eloise tried to see what the fuss was about.

'It's just a fair in the village. They do it every year. There are stalls and competitions, and Daniel has been asked to judge the pet show.' Debbie made it apparent she was delighted at the idea with her wide smile in contrast to Daniel's pursed lips.

'No. The clinic has been asked if a representative will assist. That doesn't have to be me,' he insisted.

'You're the owner and a long-term resident. It's you that they want. I can mind the clinic for a few hours.' Debbie folded her arms, preparing for battle, and Eloise imagined this was a scenario which played out frequently, both of Daniel's colleagues trying to convince him to step out into the real world every now and then.

'I don't really want to spend my afternoon drinking tea, eating home-made cake and watching pups on parade.'

'No? Sounds like my idea of heaven,' Eloise teased, wondering why he was so against it. The community was reaching out to him, keen for him to be a part of the day. If he wasn't careful, he'd become the feared local hermit instead.

'You go, then,' he said petulantly.

'Maybe I will,' she spat back. Then common sense kicked in. 'Except, no one knows who I am.'

'You could go with him, Eloise. It would be a good way for the locals to get to know you, and take some of the attention from Daniel.' It was Debbie who came up with a compromise which didn't sound like too much of a stretch for either of them.

Eloise looked over at Daniel, who began to move towards the door, ushering them all before him.

'I'll think about it,' he said, which proved sufficient to satisfy Debbie for now.

She and the receptionist waved before getting into their cars and driving off, leaving Daniel and Eloise alone. It was the first time they'd been truly on their own since that moment at her house, without their colleagues, clients or Lucky to provide a buffer. Even now, as he locked up the clinic and led her round to the house, there was a tension in the air, an anticipation that was neither justified nor wanted when she was simply holding up her end of the agreement.

'Hello, gorgeous.' Eloise was equally as thrilled to see Lucky as he was to see her, though her backside was not wiggling with quite the same enthusiasm. When she looked at him closer, however, he was not the same dog she'd left here earlier after his walk. 'Oh, Lucky. What have you done?'

'What's wrong?' Her concern drew Daniel's attention and he immediately came to her side.

'His face is all swollen.' She pointed out Lucky's muzzle, which had ballooned in size, so he looked as though he were a reflection in a funhouse mirror. It might've been comical if it didn't suggest something had happened to him.

Daniel knelt on the floor beside her to examine the dog, close enough that she could almost feel his body heat through her uniform.

'It looks like an allergic reaction to something. He didn't eat anything when you were out on your walk earlier?'

'No. He was fine when I left him. I gave him some water and left the window open so he could get some air.' She hated to think she was in some way responsible for whatever had happened to him, failing at the first hurdle as a pet owner.

'I think it's a bee sting. I see this all the time. The numpty has probably tried to eat one and got stung for his trouble. He doesn't seem to be struggling to breathe but we should take him through and give him some antihistamines.'

If there was one thing to be said about owning a pet, it was that there was never a dull moment. Certainly there was no time to sit around moping, when her thoughts were taken up with his wellbeing as much as any of her children.

The trio traipsed back into the surgery and Lucky, who looked very sorry for himself, sat quietly whilst Daniel took out a pair of tweezers to remove what was left of the stinger in his muzzle. Eloise held a cold compress to the area, trying to reduce some of the swelling.

'I think he's going to need close observation to make sure the antihistamines are doing the job. There's always a possibility of a delayed allergic reaction. Do you want me to keep him here?'

'I suppose it's for the best, but I was looking forward to having him round.' It was silly, especially in the circumstances, but she'd been longing to curl up on the sofa with the dog and a good book tonight. Just having that company made her feel safer, more comfortable, and less as though she was alone in the world.

Daniel paused, seemingly deep in thought. 'You could stay here.'

'In the clinic?' As much as she would miss having Lucky, she wasn't prepared to give up her comfortable bed for a night on the floor.

'At my house, silly.'

'Oh.'

It was a proposition she hadn't seen coming, which made her heart flip and her stomach clench. A night with Daniel was something which both appealed and terrified at the same time. The prospect would satisfy her curiosity, and more, for the man about whom she'd been having inappropriate thoughts lately.

However, she'd only ever been with her ex, and her body was entirely different from the one she'd had when they'd first met. If it had been enough to disgust a partner of over three decades, it wasn't likely to impress a new man in her life.

Daniel cleared his throat with a cough. 'I mean, I have a spare room you can stay in.'

'Of course. I knew what you meant.' She forced a nervous laugh so he wouldn't think she'd been seriously contemplating sharing his bed with him—something which apparently hadn't even crossed his mind until now.

'I just thought it might put your mind at rest. I can make us something to eat if you want to go and pack an overnight bag or something.'

Now Eloise knew he had no romantic notions towards her at all, or he wouldn't be so blasé about the matter. She knew what a big deal it would be for him to have a woman spend the night with him when he'd apparently shut himself off from the world since his wife's death. He obviously didn't think about her in any way other than as a colleague, or Lucky's co-owner. She was the one who had to get her head round the nature of their relationship and stop reading things into it that weren't there.

'I might do that. I won't be long.' Perhaps a night establishing that this was a platonic work situation would help her to get over this attraction she felt towards him. Besides, she wanted to be here for Lucky. She wouldn't rest tonight, worrying about him, worrying she might lose him before she'd even had a chance to be a dog mum.

And dinner together would just be sustenance. There was absolutely nothing to read into the fact he was cooking her a meal. And no reason to share that information with their other colleagues.

Lucky was stretched out on the bed Daniel had just made up for his overnight guest. He didn't have the heart to make him get off, and he didn't think Eloise would object. Chances were she'd spend the night with the dog cuddled up next to her anyway. She was clearly concerned about him and he could tell she'd been reluctant to leave without him. That was the only reason Daniel had made the suggestion for her to spend the night. There was no more to it than that.

As for dinner, they both had to eat, and he had food in the fridge to use up anyway. It was no big deal, even if he'd been vacuuming, dusting, and doing everything to make this room which hadn't been used in five years, comfortable for her stay in.

He and Anne had never really used it for anything even though it had been kitted out as a second bedroom. He supposed anyone else would've used it as a nursery, but since they hadn't wanted children it had never been an option. Anne had used the wardrobes to hold her overspill of clothes from their bedroom, but even they'd long ago been donated o charitable organisations. So he'd had no reason to come into this room until now, though it wasn't likely to be a regular occurrence.

'Daniel?'

He heard Eloise call from the hallway, having left the front door on the latch so she could let herself in.

'I'm just getting your room ready. Come on down.' He finished plumping the pillows, glad he'd still held onto the unopened bedding which had been in the wardrobe, intended for use in this room. It might make it seem as though he had guests over all the time, so this wasn't really a momentous occasion, even though he was already opening up parts of his life to Eloise which had been closed for a long time. He blamed the dog.

'You didn't have to go to any trouble for me.' Eloise arrived at the bedroom door, overnight bag in hand.

'It's no trouble. I think Lucky's claimed it as his room, though.' He directed her attention to the slightly less swollen dog who was now sprawled sideways across the double bed.

'I'm sure there's room enough for both of us.' Eloise plonked her things on the floor and took off her jacket to hang it on the back of the bedroom door.

Daniel was trying not to think about the fact she'd changed out of her uniform and looked much more relaxed in her jeans and loose white silk blouse. Of course she would've wanted to get out of her work clothes as soon as possible. However, it was a reminder to him that this arrangement was outside of working hours, venturing into an altogether different territory—in his spare room of all places.

'Dinner should be ready if you want to come

when you're settled.' He rushed out, not bothering to wait for her, keen to be somewhere less confined.

'What are we having?' Her voice sounded behind him as she followed him down the hallway to the kitchen.

'Nothing fancy. Just a lasagne.' Usually a whole lasagne would last him some time. Most meals he batch-cooked and froze to use at a later date. It saved him from having to shop in town every week, with supermarket deliveries not as readily available out in the countryside. At the same time, it was one step up from living off microwave meals for one, which he'd got sick of pretty quickly after Anne's death. Cooking and freezing had become part of his routine as a widower. Tonight he was sharing his food with someone for the first time in recent memory, or someone other than Lucky.

'It's more than I've managed to cook since moving here. I've been living off toasted sandwiches and instant noodles.' Without waiting for instruction, Eloise began opening the cupboards and drawers, setting their places for dinner at the table. It was as if none of this was out of the ordinary at all for either of them.

'It's better to get into a routine when it comes to cooking, before those bad eating habits are here to stay. I should know. When Anne died, I didn't see the point in cooking just for one. Sandwiches and toast were my staple for some time. I was only eating for fuel, and took no pleasure in it.'

'I wish I could say the same,' Eloise mumbled, plating up the salad he passed to her.

'You know what I mean. Grief steals away any happiness in your life. I'm just saying, don't end up like me. You still have a life to live.'

'And you don't?' Eloise looked at him with such pity in her eyes, he had to turn away.

'I had my life with Anne. I was happy. Now she's gone, and I simply have to carry on without her.' He carefully took the tray of lasagne out of the oven and cut two steaming portions, leaving the rest to cool so he could freeze it later.

'Don't you think she'd want you to be happy? I'm sure she didn't mean for you to lock yourself away from the world for ever.'

Daniel gritted his teeth as he poured them each a glass of wine to accompany their meal. This wasn't the conversation he'd expected to have over dinner. It was deeply personal and uncomfortable. Eloise was making him look at his existence through different eyes and he wasn't sure he liked what he saw.

'I've got the practice; that's all I need.'

'Did you and Anne never think about having a family?'

He shook his head. At least on that matter he could confidently defend himself. Neither he nor Anne had seen the point of bringing more lives into the world if they couldn't commit to them one hundred percent. For them, work had come first. It had been their vocation and their security. Nothing was more important than that to them. Even though Anne had grown up in a loving home with both parents, it had been a struggle for her family financially. Stability had been just as important to her as it had to Daniel—part of the reason her illness had thrown them both into turmoil. That hadn't been in their plans for their life together.

'No. We were always focused on work, and putting all of our energy into the practice. It wouldn't have been fair to have children and not give them the love and attention they deserved.' He sat down at the table with his dinner, hoping that the meal would signal the end of this particular conversation.

Unfortunately, it didn't put Eloise off. She simply carried on in between mouthfuls and compliments on his cooking prowess.

'At least you were both on the same page. It

would've been worse if perhaps you'd wanted kids and never got that opportunity. Not that either of you could ever imagine what was going to happen…' Eloise seemed to backtrack, as though she was worried she'd offended him in some way, but Daniel understood what she was getting at.

Anne's passing had left him alone in the world, which was a tragedy in itself, but he supposed if he'd wanted to be a father, and that role had been taken from him along with his wife, it would've been a double tragedy. It was bad enough being left to try and look after himself. He didn't think he would've managed it if he'd had to raise their children on his own. It would've meant more loved ones to lose further down the line too, as witnessed by Eloise's current status.

'No, but at least I'm the only one left behind.' It would've been difficult to deal with other's grief as well as his own, forced to put on a mask and carry on as though his life hadn't been completely destroyed. At least he'd been able to be his authentic self, grieving as long as he had.

'It's hard, isn't it, watching everyone carry on around you when you feel as though your life has just stopped?' Eloise was the only one he'd met who seemed to understand that. Even though her family were simply relocated elsewhere, she was grieving for the life she'd had, and lost, nonetheless.

'It can't have been easy for you. Do your daughters visit much?'

'They're very good. They call me most days to make sure I'm all right, but they have their own lives to live and adventures to enjoy. I'm happy they're doing so well for themselves and are confident enough to go out and see something of the world. I don't want them to waste their time worrying about me. I've lived my life, done the things I'd wanted to do—raised my family and had a lovely career.'

'You make it sound as though your life is over, Eloise.'

'According to everyone else, it is. My husband doesn't want me, my daughters don't need me and the rest of the world hardly knows I exist. It's not empty-nest syndrome I have. It's more like empty life. I don't seem to have a place here any more.'

'You have a place here. We want you. We need you. I'd like to think you've found somewhere here where you can start over again. You still have time.' It wasn't until he said it that Daniel realised he meant every word. He couldn't, or didn't want to, imagine Eloise moving on. She'd already become such a big part of the place, of his life, that it would seem like a huge loss if she was to leave.

It was a startling revelation about someone he'd only really known for a few weeks. If anything, he should be pleased if she suddenly decided that she wanted to move back to the city, or be closer to her daughters. Not having Eloise around would certainly make his life easier. He could return to his days and nights in which he didn't think about her. Then again, he might be lonelier than ever if she suddenly disappeared out of his life as quickly as she'd arrived in it.

'As do you.' She finished her meal and set the cutlery to one side of her plate. 'You could still bag yourself a young wife and start a family. Unlike women, men never appear to be too old to do that.'

The slight tinge of bitterness in her voice was understandable, because she was right—rock stars could go on making babies into their seventies or eighties, their wives decades younger and immeasurably prettier than their male counterpart. Not so much the other way round. For those superficial men who wanted trophy wives and families, a woman past a certain age held no appeal; once she was past child-bearing age she was of no apparent use.

But Daniel liked to think he had more substance than that. To him, a woman, or any human being, was about more than their appearance or what they could do for him. It would take a lot for anyone to live up to Anne, who'd given him a life he never thought he'd have: a house, a home, a business of his own and, more importantly, love. He would happily have spent the rest of his days with his wife, getting old and wrinkly together.

'Like I said, that's not something I'm interested in. You know, when Anne was first diagnosed, one of the first things that people said to us was how it could affect our marriage.' Like most of those afternoons spent in hospital, it wasn't one of the happier memories he had of his time with Anne, but nonetheless an important one.

'I can understand the strain it would put on a relationship. It only took something as inevitable as menopause to end mine.'

'I couldn't believe it at the time. Couldn't understand why they were telling Anne she should prepare herself for facing her treatment alone, and make arrangements for alternative support. It was insulting to me, who'd planned to be there for her every step of the way—though apparently there's an appallingly high number of men who don't stick around when their partners are diagnosed with cancer.'

Once he'd calmed down after the initial sting of what they were saying, he'd realised they were trying to prepare Anne if she had to go through chemo and surgery without him. He couldn't imagine being the sort of spineless human who ran at the first sign of trouble. As far as he'd been concerned, marriage had been for life, till death parted them.

'That's terrible. It was bad enough knowing my husband didn't care enough to see me through a few years of hot flushes and haywire hormones. I can't imagine facing difficult hospital treatment, and such an uncertain future, with someone who couldn't support me. Especially someone I've been with for a long time. Someone I've shared more than half of my life with.'

The sudden passion in her voice and pain in her eyes made him think that Eloise wasn't talking hypothetically any more. Although her circumstances were different from Anne's and his, the betrayal must've felt huge when her husband hadn't loved her enough to stick around when she'd already been feeling so low. He was the sort of man they'd been describing when they'd warned Anne to prepare for the worst.

'Honestly, it never occurred to me. I thought they were making it up when they said a high percentage of men left their wives during cancer treatment, going on to set up a new life with someone else. But apparently there are plenty who can't cope with the idea of being alone, so they plan ahead in the worst possible way.'

'But not you.' Eloise's face softened again, but he didn't want her to think he was trying to appear as some sort of martyr for sticking by his wife when she'd been sick.

'I loved her, and I never had any intention of leaving her, even when we knew she was terminal. But I wasn't afraid of being on my own either. My mother died when I was thirteen, and I was in care for most of my adolescence. I learned during those teen years not to get close to anyone. Anne was the exception. She showed me that life could be better by sharing it. It just made it all the harder when she was no longer in it.'

That pain, never far from the surface, pierced his heart deeper as he remembered the life they'd once had. One in which they'd woken up together, worked together, talked, made love and done all the other things a couple took for granted. Eloise's husband hadn't realised how lucky he was still to have her.

There was something in that moment, sharing each other's pain, exposing their grief to the other, which Eloise found cathartic. It made her realise that she wasn't just some hormonal, hysterical woman. She was entitled to feel the way she did: hard done by; abandoned; alone. Daniel had experienced those same emotions.

'I'm so sorry for everything you've been through, Daniel, but my opinion still stands. You're too young to give up on life. Hell, so am I. Maybe it's time we both stopped feeling sorry for ourselves and just put ourselves out there. We can start with judging a pet contest at the village fair. Surely that's not too scary? It's not as though I'm signing you up for a round of speed dating or something.'

Despite the fact she was trying to make light of it, the idea of setting him up with other women was something which really did not appeal to her. She had no claim over him, and he certainly didn't owe her any loyalty, but that was one area of his life she didn't want him to move on with. At least, not with someone else.

That revelation made her feel as though someone had just attached jump leads to her heart and given it an extra charge. She hadn't come here with the expectation of meeting anyone or having any sort of relationship. However, deep down, apparently she'd been harbouring something of that nature towards Daniel—a widower, clearly still grieving, who'd be horrified by the notion. Yet who still seemed to draw her closer into his life.

She jumped up from her seat as though she'd just been scalded and set to work tidying away the remains of their meal. Perhaps stepping out into the world wouldn't be so bad for either of them, expanding their horizons and their world, which sometimes only seemed to consist of the two of them and the dog.

'I'll sleep on it.' Daniel was non-committal, but at least he hadn't completely dismissed the idea.

'Thanks for dinner, but I think I'll go to bed if that's okay?' She finished loading the dishwasher and made her excuses as politely as possible.

Staying the night in his house made it impossible to put any real kind of distance between them, but at least if she went to bed now she wouldn't have to find out anything more about Daniel Grant which would only make her like him more. She was privileged that he'd opened up to her the way he had, but reaffirming the fact that he was loving and loyal wasn't going to help her stop seeing him as someone other than her boss.

'Yes, of course. Is there anything you need?' Bless him, even though she and Lucky had completely derailed whatever plans he'd had for tonight, and imposed on his hospitality, he still thought he should do more to make her feel comfortable.

Perhaps that was why these inappropriate feelings towards him had manifested in the first place. It had been so long since anyone had taken her feelings into consideration, so the slightest kindness had swept her off her feet.

'No, thank you. I'll see you in the morning.' She left him in the kitchen and hurried away, with Lucky limping after her, though she knew sleep would likely elude her. How could she hope to slumber peacefully when they were under the same roof? When her wandering mind would never let her forget the sight of him answering the door to her wearing nothing more than a towel?

Oh, she might have kept herself busy since that moment, but that didn't mean it wasn't imprinted on her psyche. She was with him when he'd said that he was attracted to people based on their character, but knowing he was as attractive on the outside as well as in his heart was a bonus. Or a curse, at least for her peace of mind.

''Night, Eloise.'

There was nothing remotely sexual in his tone, or the sleepy smile he afforded her. Yet, her body interpreted both entirely differently. Parts of her she'd thought numb, desensitised and lost for ever were coming back to life like blooms in spring. It was overwhelming to discover she might not completely have gone to seed at all. That with the right conditions she might just flourish once more.

CHAPTER SEVEN

'WHY DON'T WE just bring him with us, Daniel?'
Eloise couldn't resist those soulful eyes pleading with her to change her mind.

Lucky was just as endearing.

'Or…he could go with you and I'll stay here,'
Daniel suggested with exaggerated enthusiasm.
Sometimes he appeared much younger than his
years—playful, even. It was a side to the re-
vered vet she was sure not many got to see.
Today she was hoping to change that for both
of their sakes.

It would do him good to get out and have a
little fun, and she could use an introduction
to the rest of the village too. Maybe she could
join one of those groups that crocheted cardi-
gans and made their own jam. At least then
she'd have different hobbies than thinking about
Daniel.

'Nope. I think people might just notice. Now,
Debbie is looking after the clinic for a few

hours, so we're free to eat as much cake as we can, buy more jumble sale tat than we can ever possibly need and make someone's day by telling them their dog's cute. It's not that much of a hardship, is it?'

'I suppose when you put it like that...' Like a petulant teenager, he reluctantly grabbed his jacket and followed Lucky and her out to the car.

They'd agreed it made more sense to travel in one car to the event, and she hadn't wanted to attract more attention by suggesting they should go separately. She doubted a ten-minute drive together was going to make much difference at this point. Having dinner together and staying overnight at his house would definitely have caused a few raised eyebrows from anyone at work aware of their antics. Regardless that the only untoward things that had happened between them were completely in her imagination.

'Did you sleep okay?' he asked, once they were in the car and on their way into the village.

'Yes,' she lied. 'Thank you.'

Between thoughts of Daniel lying semi-naked—at least in her mind— a couple of rooms away, and a dog hogging most of the bed, sleep hadn't come easily. At the crack of dawn, once she'd been sure Lucky hadn't suffered any other side effects of his altercation with a bee, she'd gone home. Not before she'd run into Daniel in the kitchen, however, who'd also risen early. After refusing breakfast, and after a quick thank you and goodbye, it had been home to shower and change before coming back to work as though nothing had happened, at least from outward appearances.

Inside, she was a mess—an even bigger one than when she'd first arrived in town, only for different reasons. Now it wasn't just the fact that her husband had left her, her daughters were living their own lives away from her and that she was physically undergoing a transformation which was difficult to terms with. After last night with Daniel, and their previous interactions, her emotions were all over the place. She had to get a grip of them soon, or her new set-up here would be in jeopardy.

'Hopefully, Lucky has learned his lesson about trying to make friends with buzzy insects.' The subtext to that was that hopefully he'd never have cause to have her stay in his house again.

That was fine by her. The next time Lucky got himself in trouble, she might be inclined simply to set up camp in the clinic to keep an eye on him instead. It might feel less like crossing that line between their professional and personal lives that way.

They pulled into the Bruce Valley Community Centre car park, slowly edging past the stall owners setting up around them until they eventually got parked at the back of the small, squat building.

She made sure Lucky had his lead on securely before letting him out of the boot, leaving Daniel to lock up the car. Lucky had yet to be tested socially in an environment with lots of other dogs and she was praying he wouldn't end up causing a scene. That wouldn't do much to convince Daniel this was a good idea.

'The lady I was talking to yesterday, Mabel, said she'd meet us inside. She was thrilled that you'd agreed to do this. It was one more thing off her list, apparently, so you're her new hero.' Eloise was sure he'd be a hero for a few more people by the end of the day. He had that effect.

They walked through the car park and round the side of the building, where it was already filling up with early birds. Chattering pensioners, excited children and meandering dog walkers hovered round the entrance, waiting for the official opening. It occurred to Eloise that they probably looked like any other couple from the village out with their dog, having a nosey at what was going on today. She was sure Daniel would hate that idea, but she didn't mind someone might think she was with this lovely man. Or that he would have any interest in her.

A matronly, efficient-looking woman holding a clipboard to her ample bosom hurried over to meet them. 'Oh, Mr Grant, how lovely to see you here. I can't thank you enough for agreeing to do this. Otherwise I was going to have to do it myself, and you know I'm already judging the cake show and the gardening section. I mean, we have some guest judges, but I'm Chair of the committee, so my opinion's very important.'

'Of course. I'm honoured that you wanted me here at all. You obviously have everything in hand yourself.' Daniel pandered to the woman's sense of importance, making her blush like a school girl.

'Well, yes, but it's nice to have a new face. And you must be Eloise.' Just when Eloise thought she'd accidentally donned her invisibility cloak this morning, the woman peered at her.

'Yes, I think we spoke on the phone this morning.' Taking a not so wild guess, she'd say this was Mabel herself. She had that same efficiency, and 'no time for nonsense' attitude which had made it a very short phone call confirming that Daniel would be in attendance today.

'Indeed. Now, we're setting up the stalls inside at the minute, and the pet show isn't for another hour. I'll give you a shout when you're needed. In the meantime, enjoy the atmosphere, get yourself a cup of tea and I'll look forward to having a conflab with you later.' With that, the whirlwind which was Mabel spun off again.

Eloise looked at Daniel, who had one eyebrow raised, as if to say, *what on earth have you got us into?*

She didn't want to give him any reason to retreat, to go back to thinking that his life was better without this level of socialising, so she hooked her arm in his and directed him towards the stalls outside.

'You heard the woman. Let's go and get a cuppa. We can scout the potential winners from a distance, as long as Mabel agrees to giving us final say on the best in show. I've a feeling she doesn't defer to others easily.'

'Well, since you roped me into this, you're buying.' Daniel didn't argue, or try to shake her off as they headed to the little van selling teas and coffees, so Eloise took that as a win.

Hopefully today marked the start of them both spreading their wings a little.

'Lucky would hands-down win this if we were allowed to participate,' Eloise whispered to Daniel as the dogs were paraded in front of them.

As fond as he was of their joint charge, he couldn't bring himself to agree. Lucky was sitting obediently at their feet watching the others, tail wagging and desperate to join in, but he wasn't cover-model material. With his shaved patches, leg bandaged and still underweight, he wasn't the picture of health, even if he was a survivor. It was too bad they'd already given out the award for Pet Most Like Its Owner to the scruffy-haired guinea pig and his human counterpart who looked as though he'd just woken up. Daniel reckoned he and Eloise had a lot in common with their dog—they'd been through the wars but were still here to tell the tale.

'I think he deserves a participation rosette at least.' Daniel slipped her one of the blue ribbons they'd been handing out like candy, and she proudly attached it to Lucky's collar.

The two of them looked so pleased with themselves that Daniel couldn't help but smile at the scene. He didn't remember smiling so much until Eloise had come into his life. There hadn't been a lot to make him happy. Perhaps he'd believed he didn't deserve to smile when Anne hadn't been able to carry on with her life too. In a few weeks of being in his life, Eloise had changed that. Now, not only had he adopted a stray dog, but she'd convinced him to judge a pet show. And he was enjoying it—most likely because she was here with him.

'You've got to make a decision, Daniel,' Eloise whispered to him.

For a moment he didn't realise she was talking about picking a winner of the best dog in show, and thought she meant about her, him and whether or not he should let her into his life.

It was a bigger decision for him than choosing a husky over a dachshund. Part of him wanted that comfort, support and companionship that being with Eloise offered, not to mention the emotions she was able to rouse in him. Although having desires towards someone who wasn't his wife felt like a betrayal in itself. But Anne wasn't here, he could have another twenty or thirty years of life ahead of him and, recently, facing that alone seemed like a very dark future—even if he hadn't thought that until Eloise had come into his life.

She offered him a new way of living, a future

to look forward to. He just had to decide if he was ready for that. If he could risk the chance of getting close to someone again, when fate had a cruel way of taking everyone away from him.

Then, as Eloise nodded her head towards the eager pet owners watching him, he remembered what he was here to do. He strode forward and shook the hand of the woman who was wearing a pink bow around her neck to match that tied around her little long-haired dachshund's neck. Until that moment he hadn't known which to pick, but it had been Eloise's clear favourite. She quickly helped him distribute runner-up rosettes to those who'd made it into the final to pacify the disappointed owners.

'Congratulations on being a finalist. Thank you for participating.'

Whilst she appeased the others, Daniel found himself swamped in a hug, enveloped in a cloud of sickly-sweet perfume, the delighted winner embracing him tightly to the point where he thought he'd have to push her away so he could breathe again.

'I think the photographer from the local paper wants a photo of you and little Pixie.'

Thankfully Eloise came to the rescue, tapping the woman on the shoulder and directing her towards another man. Clearly keen to get her five minutes of fame, she unceremoniously dropped Daniel and rushed off, fixing her hair as she went.

'Thanks for that.' He could feel the heat in his face and it wasn't just from being almost smothered in someone's chest, although Eloise seemed to find his discomfort amusing, failing to hide the smirk on her face.

'I thought you might need rescuing.'

'You thought right. See, this is exactly why I don't come to these things.'

'Because women can't help but throw themselves at you?' She was teasing him, something he was used to with his other colleagues who were always trying to get him to come out of his shell. He usually didn't get drawn into it, but it was different with Eloise. He liked seeing the twinkle in her blue eyes, knowing she was getting a kick making fun of the situation. If anything, he was inclined to keep the banter going, finding his own pleasure in her enjoyment.

'Yeah, it's an awful hazard of the job. That's why I had to lock myself away at the practice. Traffic would come to a standstill, no one could get anywhere or get any work done.'

'So, really, you were doing everyone in town a favour by staying away?'

'Uh-huh. And now…'

'Everyone is being reminded of what they're missing and can't control themselves.'

'Exactly.'

'Then perhaps we should go inside before we cause a riot of stampeding admirers out here.' Eloise offered him her arm and he took it gladly. Although they were joking about a fan club, he did think people would be less likely to approach him when he was with Eloise. They presented a certain image of togetherness, which was only true because of their work relationship, but nonetheless hopefully deterred anyone approaching.

A hope which tempted fate as a harassed looking Mabel met them at the door.

'Mr Grant, can I have your assistance please? One of our contestants appears to have been in the sun too long.'

Daniel, Eloise and Lucky followed her over to a man holding a little pug in his arms. The pug was panting heavily and clearly in distress.

'Pugsley's been sick, but he won't drink any water,' the worried owner told them.

Dogs with flatter faces and shorter muzzles often had breathing difficulties, and it made them vulnerable to overheating in the warmer weather.

'The first thing we need to do is get him somewhere cool. We should take him inside. Eloise, there are cooling pads and a spray bottle. Could you get them please?' He tossed Eloise the car keys and rushed inside the community hall in search of a cooler space.

'There's a small room at the back with a fan. We can take him there.'

Mabel led them through the main hall to an office where a free-standing fan was already whirring away. Daniel suspected Mabel had been using the room in between commitments to cool herself down.

'Could we get some fresh water please?' he asked, sending Mabel off to locate it.

'Is Pugsley going to be okay? He's my daughter's dog. I'm just exercising him for her.'

'The important thing is to get him cooled down first, then we can take to the clinic for a more thorough examination. Has he had any seizures?' Daniel checked the pug's gums, the grey discoloration showing that there wasn't enough oxygen getting around his system. The excitement of the day, combined with the heat, would increase oxygen demand, resulting in the heavy panting.

'No, but he was having trouble standing.'

When Eloise returned with the cooling mat

he kept in the car for Lucky, Daniel instructed the man to set the dog down on it in front of the fan. Although they were in a cooler area now, there was still a chance that Pugsley's increased effort to breathe could cause a collapse of the inner walls around his larynx and prove fatal—a horrible way to end the day for everyone involved.

'Good boy.' Daniel stroked him slowly, speaking in a reassuring voice to encourage him to calm down as Mabel set down a bowl of water.

Eloise tied Lucky to the leg of the nearby table and began to spray the pug all over with water, letting Daniel enjoy the cooling mist drifting his way in the process.

'I think his breathing's a bit more normal now,' the pug's guardian noted, probably trying to reassure himself that everything was going to be all right.

Daniel was inclined to wait a bit longer to make sure.

'We'll probably take him back to the clinic with us to keep an eye on him.' Eloise knew as well as Daniel that damage may well have been done to the little dog's organs already. They would have to run some tests to make sure, even though he might seem fully recovered.

It was nice to have her support. Although other nurses had worked alongside him, it had been very much a job to them. They clocked in and out, their home life very separate from the clinic. Perhaps that was why he had more of a bond with Eloise, because she seemed as invested in the practice, and the patients, as he. Maybe that would change if she should ever find herself in another relationship, but she was such a kind-hearted soul he didn't think so.

It was also a disturbing thought that she might pair off with someone new and leave him behind after opening up his world. Despite telling himself not to get too close, to have her too involved in his personal life, it was too late. She was part of it now, permeating his work space and his home. He didn't want to think of either without Eloise in it.

'Would you be happy to drive us back to the clinic, Eloise? I'd like to keep Pugsley with me, just in case anything were to happen.' He wanted to have his hands free and be totally unencumbered if the little dog stopped breathing altogether and needed resuscitating.

'Of course. You could follow on behind us,' she told the man waiting anxiously beside them.

'That's fine. I want to phone my daughter

and let her know what's happening. She'll likely want to come over to see you too.'

'No problem.' Daniel took a business card out of his wallet and handed it over, before gathering Pugsley up into his arms, cooling mat and all.

This time Eloise took the lead back to the car, loading Lucky into the open boot whilst Daniel took Pugsley into the passenger seat with him. Lucky gave an excited, 'Woof!', not knowing what was going on, but clearly picking up on the charged energy in the car.

'Back to work, then,' Eloise said with a sigh, starting up the car.

She didn't have to say any more for him to know exactly what she was talking about. For a couple of hours away from reality, they'd enjoyed one another's company doing something normal, as though they didn't have any worries in the world to deal with.

A sick dog had quickly brought them back down to earth and reminded them they had a job to get back to. It also meant they would most likely see each other outside of working hours again tonight, since Eloise wasn't one to clock out just because her shift was officially over. She liked to be personally involved with the animals which might require overnight observation, echoing his work ethic and once again proving how alike they were.

It was good fortune that he'd bought extra chicken for dinner tonight when he'd probably end up cooking for two again—a routine he could find himself easily getting used to.

CHAPTER EIGHT

'YOU REALLY DIDN'T have to do this, Daniel. I could've grabbed something when I got home.' Eloise's protest was weak since she'd just finished the delicious honey soy chicken drumsticks and vegetable rice he'd presented her with for dinner.

'It's okay. I was cooking anyway, and it's nice to have company.'

Daniel cleared the dishes away and came to join her on the sofa. Lucky seemed content lying on the floor in front of the television. It was the sort of homely scene which she hadn't been part of in a long time. She knew she shouldn't get too comfortable, yet it had been lovely these past couple of nights being with Daniel, chatting over a meal together. He cared enough to include her, to think about her needs, at least when it came to dinner.

She didn't remember her ex-husband ever having done that. As a wife and mother, she'd always been the one catering for others, pandering to their wants and needs. Though she'd been happy enough to do it at the time, now she could see no one had ever really thought about her in return. And, when she'd outlived her usefulness, she'd been casually discarded. It had left a great big hole in her life which was increasingly being taken up being in Daniel's company—something which, in itself, wasn't anything to get too concerned about, except for the need now building in her to do it all the time.

'I'm glad Pugsley's going to be all right,' she said, moving them back onto work talk where it was safer.

'Yeah. You can never be too careful, but I think we got to him just in time. I suppose it's lucky we were there. I've got you to thank for that.' Daniel fixed her with his brown-eyed gaze, and Eloise felt her heart melt a little more.

'Me and Mabel,' she said with an anxious laugh, trying to deflect his gratitude.

'If it wasn't for having you by my side, Eloise, it wouldn't have entered my head to go there today—even Anne couldn't persuade me to go to things like that—but I wanted to see you having fun. It looks good on you.'

When he looked at her so intensely, said nice things to her, she was inclined to forget she was a middle-aged divorcee invisible to most people. Daniel made her believe she was someone he wanted to listen to, to be with, and she found that intoxicating. Along with the fact she was beginning to recognise herself again. She'd found a purpose here and was beginning to feel like part of the community as well as the work force.

In the mornings she'd even found herself paying a little more attention to her appearance. For a long time it hadn't seemed that important. She'd probably stopped making an effort for Sam when he never noticed anyway. At the time she'd felt too ground down by life to be bothered. Since moving here, however, she'd taken more care over how she looked. It gave her a little confidence boost, making her feel better in herself when she'd made an effort. These days she had more of a spring in her step, a reason to get up in the morning, and a lot of that had to do with Daniel.

Of course, moving here, starting over, had given her a new impetus. Here she wasn't just an abandoned wife and mother. She could start over and she wanted to make a good impression.

She liked the appreciative looks it drew from Daniel in the process, along with how it made her feel when he looked at her that way. Except now, sitting so close after an intimate dinner, she was worried her thoughts would take them somewhere neither was ready for.

'Oh, I almost forgot…' She hopped off the sofa and grabbed her bag, pulling out a little lunch box. 'Dessert.'

'Where did you get that?' He sat back and watched with interest as she lifted off the lid to reveal slices of Victoria sponge cake.

'Mabel insisted we take some home with us to thank us for helping out. I think it was from the first prize winning entry in the home baking competition.' Cake was always a good distraction, and she'd often comforted herself with a cup of tea and a slice to get those feel-good endorphins which had been otherwise missing in her life.

In this case, it was her hormones that needed some distracting… She held up a slice and, just when he was about to take a bite, she thought it would be funny to shove it in her own mouth instead. Trying not to laugh and spit crumbs everywhere, she munched on the soft sponge cake, licking the cream from her lips when she'd finished.

'Such a tease,' he said, but his deep and husky voice meant the joke had backfired on Eloise.

Far from breaking the sexual tension, she felt it even more as he watched her with hungry eyes.

Enjoying having captured his interest, she leaned into the moment. She scooped some of the cream onto her finger and held it out to him. Without hesitation, he took hold of her hand and directed her finger into his mouth. Eloise held onto her intake of breath as he slowly sucked the full length of her finger, never breaking eye contact.

This wasn't her imagination. There was something exciting happening between Daniel and her. It was both frightening and thrilling at the same time. If this went any further than a flirtation with her boss, she would risk her job, therefore her financial stability and new life here. Yet feeling this way, desirable and womanly, was something she thought she'd never experience again. It was something that might be a one-off, the last chance she might have to enjoy what was left of her femininity.

So, when he leaned forward and kissed her, she put up no resistance. They would come to their senses soon enough so she wanted to enjoy this while this moment of madness lasted.

The cake fell somewhere between them as Daniel closed the small space between their bodies, overcome with desire for Eloise. In the end he didn't know who'd been teasing who, but the inevitable outcome had been the same. His resolve—and Eloise's too, it would seem—had been stretched to breaking point.

He'd tried holding back, fighting these feelings, but he couldn't seem to stop himself. Probably because she'd given him clear signals that she was just as affected by whatever was happening between them. They hadn't been able to stay away from one another, and this kiss was the consequence of attempting to deny that attraction. All of that pent-up desire was spilling over into this hard, passionate exchange that was blowing his mind. He literally couldn't think straight when her soft lips were moulded to his, her tongue dipping into his mouth, awakening a fire that had taken him by surprise.

It was one thing discovering he was attracted to another woman who wasn't his wife, but he hadn't expected the chemistry to completely take over. All those doubts he'd had about giving into his urges, the thoughts of how it would be a betrayal of his wife's memory, were drowned out by the sound of his blood rushing in his ears. One kiss had made him realise how stale his life had become, and he was reluctant to go back to that situation any time soon.

'Stay with me tonight,' he muttered against her lips.

'In the spare room?' she asked, those big, blue eyes questioning his true intention.

'No…with me.' Daniel needed to be honest with them both about what he wanted. Then perhaps one of them would use the opportunity to come to their senses.

He watched her gulp, saw the slight panic in her eyes and realised this was as big a deal for her as it was for him. 'Is that a good idea?'

'Probably not.' He made them both smile nervously, but neither of them could look away from the other.

In the end he was the one to take the initiative, getting to his feet and taking her by the hand.

Eloise followed him as he led her to his bedroom, the place where he'd spent every night on his own for the past five years.

'We don't have to stay here. We could go into the other room if you'd prefer?' Eloise apparently understood the significance of him bringing her in here, but he didn't want her to read more into this than it being any more than a much-needed release for both of them.

He shook his head. 'No. I have to move on some time.'

It was becoming obvious that he couldn't spend the rest of his days alone. He wasn't a saint. And, though he'd loved Anne, his feelings hadn't died with her...as his body was strongly reminding him.

He knew he wasn't ready for a serious commitment, but surely he deserved some happiness? It had been in short supply for over five years. And being with Eloise made him happy.

'You're shaking.' He reached out to a trembling Eloise and pulled her into his embrace.

Having her soft form pressed against his revitalised all sorts of emotions inside him. It was comforting and arousing at the same time. His body and his mind were in tandem for once, wanting this, needing Eloise.

'It's been a long time since I've done this with anyone. I've only ever been with my husband, and I... I'm not exactly in my first flush of youth.' She was mumbling into his chest, as though she was too embarrassed to look him in the eye.

Daniel released his hold a little so he could lift her chin up and make her look up at him. 'You're beautiful.'

He dropped a soft kiss on her mouth and she began to relax into him again. It was reassuring to know that they were both venturing into unfamiliar territory, even though he was under pressure to make it good for both of them. This needed to be worthwhile, since they were going against their better judgement.

Eloise's hands were pressed against his chest, her body heat branding him with her touch, and he was suddenly desperate for that skin-on-skin contact. It was a long time since anyone had touched him.

He undid the first few buttons of his shirt, then pulled it over his head in impatience, eliciting a smile from Eloise. The look of appreciation she gave as she swept her gaze over his body did wonders for his self-esteem. Like her, he had some reservations about getting older, his physique not the same as the last time he'd been with a woman. As she traced her hands over his chest, his stomach and down to the waistband of his trousers, it appeared he'd passed muster.

'Is it sore?' she asked, when she grazed over the vivid bruises left from his accident in her house.

'Not now,' he said; he wasn't aware of anything except the feel of her on his skin.

Daniel sucked in a breath when she undid the button and let his trousers fall to the floor. The graze of her fingers below his waist made him tingle all over in delicious anticipation of that touch everywhere else.

'Someone's been working out.' Her honeyed voice was appreciative and laden with lust, increasing his own arousal.

'Just swimming in the loch.' A cold-water dip was his reminder he was still alive. It connected him with the world every morning and helped him forget his troubles for a little while as he focused on regulating his breathing. It wasn't something he did to impress anyone. Though he was currently reaping the benefits of Eloise seeing the results of his early-morning routine.

'Mmm, maybe I should try it.'

'I'd like that. Though you'd have to wear a lot less clothes than you're wearing now.'

'Oh, really?' Her eyes were shining as he began undoing the buttons on her blouse.

'Yeah. I mean, this top would only weigh you down.' He slipped it off her shoulders, revealing her white lacy underwear.

'And the jeans?'

'Have to go, obviously.' He unbuttoned them and slowly pulled down the zip. Just before he was able to push them over her hips, Eloise grabbed hold of his hands with hers.

'Wait,' she said, panic in her eyes, and sudden tension in her body.

'What's wrong?' As much as he wanted this, Daniel would stop the second she decided it wasn't what she wanted after all. This would only work if they were both in the moment.

'I've had two children, I eat too much cake… I'm embarrassed about the idea of getting naked in front of you.' She had her arms wrapped around her belly, trying to hide it from him. Which, in the circumstances, might seem absurd, except he knew something about those anxieties.

He had his own insecurities about aging; he didn't know anyone who didn't. Going grey, losing hair, not being as fit or toned as he used to be, were all superficial things he thought about these days when faced with an older reflection in the mirror. None of which changed him as a person.

'We're all a little softer around the middle. It doesn't make you any less beautiful to me, Eloise.' He kissed the side of her neck, nuzzling into the crook of her shoulder, and heard her suck in a shaky breath.

As he made his way across her decolletage, dropping tiny kisses, he felt her begin to relax beneath him. He carefully peeled her hands away from her stomach and she let them drop to her sides. It was a sign of her trust in him that she was being so vulnerable in front of him, exposing her insecurities and hoping he wouldn't shame her the way her husband apparently had.

Not that he could see any reason why she should've been subjected to such treatment. Her soft white skin smelled of raspberries and cream and tasted just as sweet on his tongue. He cupped the mounds of flesh rising from her lacy bra and swept his tongue over one, then the other. She gasped when he undid the clasp and released her voluptuous breasts to his gaze. Daniel plucked her nipples between his fingers until they were tight pink buds ripe for the taking. He flicked his tongue over one tip, enjoying Eloise's little moan of pleasure in response. And when he sucked her into his mouth, grazed his teeth over the sensitive nub, her body seemed to melt against him.

'Can…can we take this slow?' She gasped. 'It's been a long time.'

'Sure. We don't have to rush anything. I want you to enjoy it, Eloise.'

His own body was throbbing with need, and he was severely testing his own restraint, but for Eloise's sake he needed to take his time. He took her by the hand and led her over to the bed, feeling just as nervous as she looked. It had been a long time for him too. Hell, he hadn't even realised he still had such urges when he'd focused all his time and attention on work for the past five years. He thought his libido had died alongside his wife. Since Eloise had entered his life, he'd learned differently. He was still a man with needs and wants. All of which apparently included Eloise.

'Are you okay?' he asked as they lay down together.

Eloise bit her lip as she nodded. 'It's just… I don't know how it's going to feel, for you, or me. You hear all these stories about menopause and how it ruins your sex life. I'm afraid it's not going to be good.'

Daniel understood her fears. He'd been through this with Anne, but there were always ways to make sex enjoyable for both parties. 'I'm sure it'll be fine. We'll take our time, and if something doesn't feel right just let me know. Okay?'

'Okay.'

He silenced her doubts with a hard kiss until she was limp beneath him, totally lost to him. It was a powerful position and one he wouldn't abuse. He began his journey down her body again, kissing, licking and tasting every inch of skin he came into contact with, though when he nudged her legs apart he felt her tense again.

'So beautiful,' he mumbled, kissing the soft skin of her inner thighs, feeling her heat as he licked his way up to her most intimate area.

Eloise let out a small cry but, when he looked up to make sure she was okay, her eyes were closed, her head thrown back, and she clearly enjoyed what he was doing, confirmation that he should continue his endeavours.

He parted her legs, opening her up to him, and lapped her with the flat of his tongue. She trembled beneath him and reached down to tangle her fingers in his hair. With the tip of his tongue he dipped inside her, circling and teasing that swollen sweet spot and making her arch off the bed. Provoking such an immediate, responsive reaction to his intimate touch made him wonder what either of them had worried about. Eloise's arousal was as obvious as his own and, the more she clenched around him, writhed beneath him, the harder he fought to bring her to that final release.

The sharp pain as she tugged his hair was of no consequence compared to the feeling of pride inside as he brought her closer to orgasm. And when she cried out, bucked against him, and let her climax claim both of them, Daniel felt like the king of the world. He'd made her feel good and hopefully brought her some happiness, as well as a sense of achievement for both of them.

'Thank you,' Eloise said breathlessly when Daniel moved back up the bed to lie beside her again. Words could never convey the gratitude she felt towards him for what he'd just done, but it was all she could do for now. Her body was limp from his attentions, unused to the exertion of an orgasm which seemed to have come from her very soul, as though she'd been waiting a lifetime for the release.

Maybe she had. She didn't remember sex with Sam ever prompting such an overwhelming reaction from her body—a body she'd thought incapable of giving her, or anyone else, any satisfaction ever again. Boy, had she been wrong! If she never ever felt this way again, at least she'd have the memory to cling on to for ever: this contented, self-satisfied, cat-that-got-the-cream happiness that Daniel had gifted her.

'Are you okay?' he asked, watching her intently, his concern for her evident.

Everything about the moment made her want to weep with joy, not least the discovery that she wasn't the dried-up old hag she feared she'd

become. A life, a sex life, was still possible beyond divorce and menopause. She would never
have known that if it weren't for Daniel.

He'd taken his time to make sure she was
comfortable, at the same time making her so hot
for him she'd been on the edge before he'd even
touched her. There was a passion inside her that
she hadn't known existed until now. Until recently, sex with her husband had been routine
and familiar. Even kissing Daniel was exciting, inciting feelings in her that made her feel
shiny and new, much younger than her forty-
nine years.

In a lot of ways she felt like a born-again
virgin. It was an absurd notion for a divorced
mother of two, but she was discovering herself
again, along with her new-found sexuality. The
day might come when she didn't have the same
urges, but until then she was going to enjoy everything Daniel had awakened inside her.

'For now.' She leaned over and kissed him,
stroking a hand down his body, keen to give
him the same high she was still coming down
from.

The stomach Daniel had tried to persuade her
had become soft over the years was tight as he
flexed at her touch. He gave a sharp intake of

breath as she ventured lower and took hold of his long length, then a satisfied grin.

'You're playing with fire…' He growled, his voice hoarse with desire.

'You're the one who lit the match,' she reminded him. He'd been the one to cross that line when he'd kissed her and started this chain reaction.

His mouth tightened into a thin line, and his eyes fluttered shut as she moved her hand along his shaft. She was enjoying watching him fight for control, knowing that she could make him feel this way, that he was responding to her touch as though she was desirable after all.

As he had done to her, she flicked her tongue over his nipple, watching with glee as the flat disc grew taut with arousal. Before she had an opportunity to tease him any further, Eloise found herself flat on her back, Daniel on top of her. The weight of his body on her was as welcome as his passionate kisses. It felt right, like something she hadn't known she'd been missing in her life.

With her arms wrapped around his neck, she lost herself in those kisses. They were something that might seem unimportant to most people, but was so intimate to Eloise. It was a deep, personal connection, something more than simply the physical act of sex itself. She didn't even know if she would feel this way with anyone else, or if this was merely 'Daniel lust' that had overtaken her body and brain.

'Hold on. We still need some contraception.' Daniel's voice was urgent in her ear, his restraint clearly stretched to breaking point and fuelling Eloise's desire with that knowledge. He reached into his nightstand and took out a packet of condoms.

'I bought these when I was doing the shopping. An impulse buy, just in case. I hadn't planned this.' He seemed embarrassed by his foresight but at this moment in time Eloise was glad of it.

'At least in the future it won't be such an issue. There are some perks to this menopause lark.' Not that there'd be any way of knowing if he'd still want to do this with her when that time came.

Although she was only in the early stages of menopause, it had felt like the beginning of the end: the knowledge that she wouldn't be able to conceive another child, the death of her femininity. Even though she'd never imagined having any more babies, that choice being taken away from her seemed a cruel reminder that she was no longer useful as a woman simply because she'd got older. Thankfully she was making peace with that aspect of the aging process.

Daniel didn't need any further persuasion. He tested her readiness first, dipping his finger inside her and starting that pulsing need for him all over again. She was slick with arousal when he joined their bodies together, but that first contact still took her breath away.

'Daniel...wait...' It felt like losing her virginity all over again, and she needed a moment to adjust and accommodate him.

'What's wrong?' His genuine concern for her was there in his eyes and the tone of his voice. Knowing he cared for her was enough to help her relax a little.

'I just need a second or two to get used to you,' she explained.

'Is there anything I can do to make this easier for you?'

'Just kiss me.' It was ironic that, despite their bodies being forged together, she still needed that extra element of intimacy, that proof that he wanted *her*, not just anyone.

Daniel took his time kissing her thoroughly, teasing and tasting, showing her a tender regard that almost brought her to tears. This was more than sex, though she knew neither of them would admit it. They were discovering themselves, as well as each other. Eloise wasn't sure she would've been able to do this with anyone else, but Daniel made her feel safe... wanted...appreciated. All things that had been missing in her life too long. It wasn't long before she was a puddle of need wanting more... wanting Daniel.

He waited until she relaxed again, then moved slowly until she got used to the sensation of him inside her. He filled her again and again, driving Eloise to that pinnacle of ecstasy she'd thought she'd never reach again. Every thrust, every groan, was interspersed with tender kisses, reassuring her that he was interested in more than his satisfaction, though she knew this was about more than a physical release for him too.

This was a lot more than a casual hook-up for both of them, regardless that they were reluctant to commit to anything. Even tonight hadn't been planned. Their libidos had apparently taken over, bypassing all those red flags of warning that this wasn't a good idea.

It didn't matter that he was her boss still mourning his wife, or that she was grieving her losses too, when they could make each other feel this good. And why was that such a bad idea anyway? Who said there had to be more to this than enjoying the pleasure there was to be had sharing a bed? They weren't doing anything wrong, and it felt so right she didn't want it ever to end, because then they'd have to go back to the real world and remember why they'd been trying to avoid this for so long.

All the superficial things she'd worried so much about didn't seem important when Daniel was made love to her, making her feel so good. It could get addictive, this enjoyable reminder that she could still be sexual, desirable. Not to mention this building arousal she knew was about to carry her away onto a cloud of bliss.

'Don't stop!' she cried, as he pushed her ever closer to the edge. And, when he growled her name, he pushed her right over. Her orgasm claimed her completely; that out-of-body experience as her soul seemed to drift above her body was a euphoria she hadn't known in an age, and she never wanted to come back down from it.

When Daniel's climax followed soon after hers, it seemed to last an age. The accompanying cry made it sound as though he'd been waiting a lifetime for that release. He crashed down on the bed beside her, both of them grinning and panting for breath.

'I'd forgotten how good that felt.' Eloise

wasn't sure it ever had been that amazing with Sam. Daniel seemed to bring out the best in her, in every way possible.

'Me too.' At least he knew what she was going through. Both of them had ventured out of their comfort zone together. It had made it easier for her to admit she was nervous and ask him to make concessions for her.

The care Daniel had taken with her to make sure she was comfortable helped her relax, made her know she was safe with him. It wasn't just his own pleasure he cared about, and that went a long way to making her feel at ease with him.

'Thanks, Eloise.' He leaned across and kissed her, making her heart flutter all over again.

It might have seemed an odd thing to thank someone after sex, except she felt the same thing: gratitude; thankfulness for sharing this experience, letting her know it was still possible to have a satisfactory sex life. More than that, to enjoy great sex.

It was going to be difficult working alongside one another, knowing that this was possible together. For two people who'd been isolated, locked in their own worlds for so long, it was a revelation to find there could be something good again in their lives. Eloise just didn't know if Daniel was ready to accept it, or her, on a long-term basis.

CHAPTER NINE

DANIEL FELT AS though he'd just been hit by a truck. His body was completely spent, and the air had been knocked from his lungs. He didn't remember ever feeling this way after sex, and he didn't think it was just down to his age or the fact he'd been celibate for five years.

This was all about Eloise. About how she made him feel, and how he'd just been able to fully express that. It was where they went from here that was going to be the sticking point.

'Well, that was…'

'Unexpected? Amazing?' Eloise offered when he was at a loss to describe what had just happened.

'Both of those things.' He couldn't take his eyes off her naked body as she gave a languid stretch, providing him with a perfect view of her full figure. He couldn't resist kissing her again, as though marking his territory. For a little while, here in his bed, she was his.

His sex life with Anne had been great, but never so exciting. It was difficult to process his feelings about that when it felt so disloyal to admit it. He wondered if the reason they'd stayed together so long was because he'd been grateful to her for loving him. She'd provided the security he craved, but their relationship hadn't had the same passion he'd just shared with Eloise.

'Do you want me to go?'

'What? No.' The thought of her going now, leaving him alone and perhaps never getting to feel this way again, was something he didn't want to contemplate—at least, not yet.

'I just… I didn't think you'd want anyone to see me leaving in the morning.'

'We've got plenty of time before then. Besides, I don't know about you, but I'm not sure I can even walk at the minute.' His legs were still trembling, his heart pounding and he'd never felt so alive.

'Probably not!' She laughed, then moved over to cuddle into his side.

Daniel wrapped his arm around her shoulder, her head on his chest, and pulled the covers up over their bodies. It was a cosy picture he'd never thought he'd get to be part of again. The contentment of lying in this bed with Eloise was a snapshot he would keep in his heart for ever.

The logical part of his brain, which was just about working, knew she would have to go. They couldn't afford their colleagues to see them together, because that would mean labelling what this was, and that was a step too far just now. However, he wanted to enjoy this moment of peace for as long as possible before the guilt and doubt had time to kick in.

'I never expected this to happen, you know. It's not why I made dinner.' Although, he knew he'd had Eloise in mind when he'd been shopping for the ingredients, knowing dinner would be all the better if he had her to share it with. He hadn't been wrong.

'I know. I didn't even know it was possible— for me, I mean. I don't know what's happening with my body any more...' Eloise's feeling of powerlessness was obvious, and he felt for her. It was bad enough that he didn't seem to have control over his emotions; he could only imagine how it was for her, being a slave to her hormones.

'I know menopause was tough for Anne too. Then we had the cancer diagnosis, and she had to go through chemo too.'

He didn't know if it was insensitive of him to

mention his wife after sex with another woman, but he wanted Eloise to know he understood a little of what she was going through. Anne had gone through the mood swings, the sweats and the irregular periods, and he'd seen how she'd suffered. He'd been there to support her through it all, but at the time she'd described it as her body betraying her.

'Menopause is awful. Sorry, I know she went through so much more than me, but still, it sucks. At least I have my two girls. Sorry, that's insensitive of me...'

'It's okay. Children were never on our agenda.'

'Even so, I'm sure Anne struggled with the fact that her chance to be a mother had been taken away from her. We never intended to have any more children either, but that doesn't mean I'm not mourning the loss of my femininity.'

Daniel had never looked at it that way. He'd only seen the physical symptoms and the toll they'd taken on Anne. She'd certainly never mentioned feeling less of a woman when her periods had finally stopped. He supposed she'd been saving him from knowing how much she was suffering on the inside as well as outwardly. It didn't bring him any peace, knowing that.

'You certainly didn't seem any less of woman to me.' He skimmed his hand over the indent of her waist and her hips, luxuriating in her curves.

'It was a surprise to me too. I didn't think I'd ever get to enjoy this again. I mean, this could be a one-off for me—a last hurrah before everything south packs up shop for good. If that's what happens, then I'm glad we've had this tonight.' Eloise reached up and stroked his cheek. He caught her hand and kissed her palm.

'It's not the end of the world, you know. There is treatment: hormones and patches and whatever. You'll get back on an even keel.'

'I haven't had the chance to see a GP yet with trying to sort out the house, so I've still to look into all my options, but it'll never be quite the same, will it?'

Daniel was beginning to see why she'd worried so much. Her future was uncertain, unknown, and he knew how terrifying that could be. All he could do for now was help her enjoy this time together before everything changed.

'We could test that theory…'

'You mean…?'

'I'm game if you are.' He reached for her again, pulling her flush against his body.

She wasn't the only one who'd worried about age catching up with the body. He wasn't the young man he used to be, but thankfully a certain part of him was still able to recover quickly.

'Oh, I'm game. As long as you don't mind me being the games master.' To his surprise, Eloise rolled him onto his back and straddled his lap. Daniel's arousal immediately reached full throttle.

'I'm all for equal opportunities.' He grinned, gripping her hips as she moved against him.

She took control, impaling herself on his erection, making them both gasp at the sudden, intimate connection. Although she felt amazing around him, her new-found confidence was equally thrilling. From someone who'd been afraid to let him see her naked, she was now riding on top, free from inhibition.

If this was the effect one round of love-making had on her, he was content to keep going long into the night. She needed to have a higher opinion of herself, one that matched his own. Eloise was an amazing woman, and clearly not enough people had told her that lately. This seemed more like the real Eloise. The one who hadn't been worn down by life and an unappreciative husband. Her hands were braced on his chest and she was seeking her own satisfaction, taking him with her on the ride.

He watched the ecstasy on her face, felt her

tighten around him as her climax built, and when she let go he went with her. That feeling of complete release and peace was something he'd never tire of, yet something he'd denied himself for a long time.

He knew if roles had been reversed, and Anne had been the one left behind, he would have wanted her to find happiness again. As far as he was concerned though, for him that would always bring unhappiness somewhere else down the road. The danger of getting too used to this, enjoying being in a relationship again, was another risk of losing someone who meant a lot to him. Even though Eloise wasn't suffering from a terminal illness, the fact that he was her boss, and she had baggage of her own to deal with, brought different challenges. If being together made things difficult at work, she might decide to move on somewhere else, and that would still mean losing her.

Yet, he knew they would both benefit from continuing to see each other. They were able to remind one another that their lives hadn't ended. Perhaps some time together getting used to being in one another's company would open them up to the possibility of another relationship in the future, even if it wasn't with each other.

Right now, he wasn't sure they were able to commit, or provide the sort of long term stability they needed to move on from their past. That didn't mean he was willing to give up this new, exciting development in discovering more about Eloise and himself. They both needed, and deserved, to have this sort of intimacy in their lives. He hoped this wasn't the one-off she'd suggested, but the start of their exploration together, of finding out about the needs and desires that had been lying dormant and had awakened with a roar.

However, this could only work if they kept their private life separate from work, if they kept things physical without letting their hearts get in the way. He had to go back to being the Daniel he'd been before he'd met Anne, and shut himself off emotionally from anything that might come back to hurt him. He only hoped it wasn't already too late.

When Eloise woke up and reached over to the other side of the bed, all she found was an empty space. For a moment her sleep-addled mind wondered where she was…if she'd forgotten she'd gone home at some point. She'd expected to find Daniel lying next to her. In fact, she'd looked forward to waking up next to him.

Then she looked around the room, at the unfamiliar aqua-green coloured walls and the pine bedroom furniture, and realised she was still in Daniel's bed. He just wasn't here with her.

She couldn't believe the sense of loss she felt already, after just one night with him. After years of separate rooms, even before the divorce, she should be used to sleeping on her own. It was just nice to have someone there again, making her feel safe and wanted. Not to mention that power she'd felt, driving him out of control with lust for her. Being with him had helped her rediscover the old Eloise who didn't have to worry about her weight, medical problems or the distance between her family and her. She'd actually been able simply to enjoy her time with Daniel.

'Morning.' He appeared from the bathroom brushing his teeth, already dressed.

Although her heart sped up at the sight of him, she couldn't help the sense of disappointment that their time together had apparently come to an end. She glanced at the digital clock on the nightstand. It was only six a.m., but he was making it clear he wanted her gone.

'Morning.' Her response was half as enthusiastic as his as she threw back the covers and began retrieving the clothes that had been discarded over the floor last night in the heat of their passion. She supposed her body needed the rest several times over, unused to its exertions. However, she was reluctant to go in case she never had this experience again.

Once Daniel had finished in the bathroom, she ran in, clutching her clothes to her naked body. She wasn't quite so bold in the cold light of day. 'I won't be long.'

Without her own toiletries to hand, she had to make do with soap and water to freshen up, and a squirt of toothpaste on her finger in place of a toothbrush. At least if Daniel was insistent on her going home she'd have time to shower and change before work, though she was a bit miffed she wasn't even being offered breakfast. Okay, so it might be a one-time deal, but they still had to see each other. This wasn't some anonymous hook-up with someone he was never going to cross paths with again. His attitude was the equivalent of phoning her a taxi to get rid of her as soon as possible.

'I guess I'll be on my way.' When she came out of the bathroom, Daniel was sitting on the edge of the bed, waiting. She didn't want to make this any more awkward than it already was when they were going to have to work together in another couple of hours. Goodness knew how she was supposed to carry on as though last night had never happened when it had completely rocked her world. He'd made her think about what she was missing out on, and if it was possible she might not have to spend the rest of her life on her own after all.

'I—I thought you might like to go swimming with me this morning.' He was fidgeting with his hands, not quite meeting her eye, as though he was asking her out on a first date and they hadn't spent most of last night naked together.

'Swimming? Like, in the loch? What about work?' She couldn't have been more shocked if he'd asked her to stroll into town hand in hand. At least he wasn't trying to get rid of her, so she hoped that meant he wasn't harbouring any regrets about sleeping together. She certainly wasn't.

'We've got plenty of time. I thought we could swing by your place so you could get your swimming things, then head down to the loch. I've made us some tea to take with us.'

It was such a sweet gesture, Eloise was going to ignore the fact that taking an ice-cold dip at this ungodly hour was the last thing she'd ever want to do. Daniel was extending their time alone together and she wasn't going to turn that down. Especially if it meant they might have a chance to continue whatever it was happening between them.

'Sure. What about Lucky?' She didn't want to neglect the other man in her world.

'I've already taken him for a walk. As soon as his leg is healed, he'll be able to go swimming too, but in the meantime I think we should keep him away from the water.'

'I didn't even hear you leave.' Eloise tried not to get too excited about the prospect of this morning routine becoming a full-time arrangement if he was talking about taking the dog once he was healed. Of course, he could be talking about going solo, but why else mention it if he wasn't going to include her?

And this was why she needed to stop reading things into everything he said…

'You were out for the count and I didn't want to wake you. You looked so peaceful. Besides, I kept you up late last night.' His eyes took on that dark, hungry glaze that made her pulse flutter, along with every other part of her.

The mere mention of what they'd been up to into the small hours of the morning made her want to do it all over again. However, with Daniel up and dressed before she'd awakened, it gave a clear indication that he wasn't ready for that. She didn't want to push things too far when she didn't even know what it was she wanted herself. An affair with the boss didn't seem like the smartest move for someone just starting out, and if it turned out to just be a one-time thing it might be easier for them to move past.

'I guess we should go, then, if we want to have time for that cuppa before work?' The sooner they got out of this bedroom, the less likely they were to submit to temptation again. Then they might be able to think a bit clearer about what happened next and what they wanted from one another.

Eloise was almost giddy as they pulled up outside her house. It reminded her of her teenage years when she'd been excited about Sam coming to take her out to the cinema, or an early-bird dinner at the local restaurant.

She rushed upstairs and rifled through her drawers. It took her a while to locate her black one-piece swimsuit. She hadn't worn it in an age, since she'd become paranoid about her rounded tummy. Although she enjoyed swimming, she'd become stuck in that vicious circle—not wanting to be seen in public in anything but baggy clothes, yet the lack of exercise adding to her weight problem. Here it didn't matter, since Daniel had seen her in a lot less and hadn't complained. He'd actually been very complimentary, but she didn't think anyone here was ready for skinny-dipping just yet.

'It's so peaceful here.' As they got out of the car in the layby near the loch, the only sound was the early morning birds chirping in the trees and the rustle of leaves in the breeze.

'That's why I like to come here first thing. It sets me up for the day. Puts me on an even keel before the madness of barking dogs and hissing cats.'

She supposed it was a big adjustment every day, transitioning from the quietness of being in his house alone into the bustling veterinary practice. Eloise, on the other hand, longed for that busy white noise that came with running a family home.

Whilst she didn't miss the city so much, she wasn't used to living on her own like Daniel. She'd gone straight from living with her parents to being married, then being a housewife and mother. It had seemed like a punishment to have all of that taken away from her when she'd spent years looking after everyone else. Maybe she could learn something from Daniel and find the peace she was searching for here.

He took a bag and blanket from the boot of the car and led her down the bank via a small trail where the grass had been trodden flat, most likely worn down from his routine morning swim. Daniel seemed like a creature of habit, which made it all the more remarkable that he was including her.

'It's going to be cold at first, but your body will soon adjust.' He began stripping off, folding his clothes into a pile as he went.

Eloise tried not to stare as she undressed. Somehow it seemed more intimate to strip off here together in the broad daylight, even though they weren't planning anything more than an early morning dip.

Daniel waded into the water first, giving her a quick glimpse of his cute backside in his swimming shorts, before turning to wave her in. It was tempting to rush in so he didn't get a good look at her in her swimsuit, but the moment she stepped into the water the cold took her breath away.

'It's freezing!' She kept her arms and chest out of the water as much as she could, walking out to meet him.

'You'll get used to it. Just take deep breaths.' He held her hands and coached her through some breathing exercises.

Eloise tried to follow his instruction but she couldn't get past the pain the icy water caused every exposed part of her. It was like needles jabbing at her skin.

'Tell…me…why…this…is…a…good…idea…' It was difficult to get the words out in between gasps of air.

'It's good for the heart—increases circulation. And it wakes you up in the morning.'

'Well, one of those things is true…' She was standing on her frozen tiptoes, trying to keep as much of her body out of the water as possible.

'It's better to just dive in there so your body adjusts to the temperature.' Daniel started by splashing some water on his face and chest, then threw himself onto his back and lay there floating, daring her to do the same.

Eloise could never be called a coward. With a deep breath, she bent her knees and ducked her head right under the surface so she was completely submerged in the cold depths of the loch. It wasn't long before she sprang up again, gasping for air, since it all seemed to have left her lungs. At this stage, though, she had nothing else to lose, so she launched herself forward, keeping her head up, letting her arms and legs propel her towards Daniel.

'See? You'll get used to it,' he said, rolling over onto his belly before swimming away.

'I'm not so sure about that,' she grumbled, unconvinced about the benefits, or the enjoyment he claimed to associate with the experience.

What she did know was that she was doing it to spend more time with Daniel, and that said something about the strength of feeling she had towards him. She wasn't usually the sort of person who'd feign interest in anything to keep someone else happy—at least, not any more.

When she realised that was the reason she'd stayed in her marriage so long, she felt like a fraud. She might have got out sooner, made a different life for herself before she got too old for it, if she hadn't simply tried to play the good wife for far too long. If she'd been honest with her husband and herself, they might've parted ways a long time ago. She supposed she should be thankful to him for finally having the courage to end it for her. Despite how hurt she'd been, it was probably better in the long run to go their own ways than to pretend they still had a relationship. Eloise didn't want to pretend any more.

After a few laps up and down, doing her best

to take in the beautiful scenery and quietness, she had to admit defeat.

'Sorry, Daniel. I'm going to have to get out. It's just too cold for me.'

The look of disappointment on his face was apparent, but she knew it was only because he wanted her to enjoy it as much as he did. As she dried off, wrapping a huge towel around her body, he began to emerge from the water too. His skin pink, his hair plastered to his scalp and swimming shorts moulded to him, he was a sight worth coming here for.

'You don't have to get out of the water because of me. I'm happy to sit here and warm up.' *And watch.*

'It's fine, just a quick dip. I'm not a masochist!' He grinned, and she was glad she was forgiven for prematurely ending the swim session.

'Here. You need to get warmed up too.' She handed him another towel, watching as he dried his hair and body before doing a quick change beneath it. The logistics of changing out of her wet things and into her work clothes was a little trickier for her, trying not to flash her bits to unsuspecting hikers who might happen by. Somehow she managed it, just about keeping her dignity intact.

'This will help get some heat back into us.'

Daniel rummaged around in the bag and pulled out a small metallic flask and two cups. He poured them both a cup of hot, steaming tea, then produced a spread of croissants, muffins and fresh fruit.

Now this was more like it.

'Do you do this every morning?'

'Pretty much. Although, I've put on a bigger breakfast spread than usual for you.' He took a huge bite of a croissant, flaky crumbs dropping onto the stubble of beard lining his strong jaw.

Eloise supposed it wouldn't be appropriate to lick them off. Instead, she made do with a blueberry muffin, breaking it into small pieces before eating it so she didn't make a mess, even though she was ravenous. Exercise was certainly making her hungry. Between great sex and swimming, she was getting more of a workout than usual and she had to admit she did feel great.

'It's very much appreciated.' She washed the cakey goodness down with some hot tea, slowly beginning to thaw from the inside out.

'So, wild swimming isn't for you, then?' She wasn't clear if he was asking out of politeness or if it was more of an open invitation to join him again. Eloise wasn't going to turn down a chance to spend more quality time with him.

'I could *learn* to love it. It is invigorating, and I'm definitely wide awake now.' She could see why it appealed to Daniel, but having breakfast together was the bit she was enjoying the most. It was a reward for her effort, and that was definitely something she could get used to.

'I could stay here all day.' Daniel sighed and stretched out flat on the blanket, hands behind his head and eyes closed.

Eloise acted instinctively, leaning over to kiss him. It was a thanks for everything he'd done for her last night and this morning. It was also an urge she couldn't seem to pass up when she looked at him, which was going to make work interesting.

She knew was taking a chance by continuing what had happened last night into today. They hadn't discussed how they wanted to play this: if it was a spontaneous event which should be consigned to the past, or perhaps was the start of something for them. However, since he'd been the one to suggest she join him this morning, she was willing to take the chance that he hadn't tired of her already.

It was one that paid off, as Daniel slipped his arms around her neck and pulled her deeper into the kiss. Only when she began to get a crick in her neck because of the awkward angle she sat at did she break away. 'I wasn't sure if you still wanted that.'

'Did it feel like I didn't want that?'

'You know what I mean, Daniel. What is it exactly we're getting into?' She wanted to be clear from the outset so she wouldn't be blindsided when he dumped her like everyone else. At least if she was aware this feeling of being wanted had a shelf life, she might better be able to prepare for it this time.

He sat up and hugged his knees. 'I have no idea.'

'Helpful.'

At least she made him laugh.

'I'm sure neither of us planned for this to happen, and maybe that's the way we should continue.'

'Aimlessly?' She wasn't sure if that was enough for her. Being held at his whim, waiting for word if he still wanted her or if he'd decided she wasn't worth the hassle of adjusting his lifestyle to include her, was a precarious position she'd been in once too often already. He screwed up his face at that description. Her whole new life, possibly her future, was riding on how this worked out.

'I understand how big of a deal this is, moving on from Anne, and I don't want to put you under any pressure to make a decision. However, I'm a little concerned about where this would leave me in terms of my job if you decide this isn't what you want—that I'm not want you want.'

She swallowed hard. It was difficult to admit that was what was going on inside her head when it sounded so desperate, so needy, but she needed some clarification, some reassurance she hadn't just screwed everything up when she'd started to settle in here.

He was frowning by the time she'd finished. 'One thing I can assure you of is that I intend to keep my work and personal life separate. I always have—until now, at least. If we'd met anywhere else, this wouldn't even have entered your head. Whatever happens between us, your job is safe. I think we're both old enough and wise enough to figure out the important things in life.'

Eloise wasn't so sure when they'd already failed to acknowledge that last night had probably changed everything for them, but she didn't argue as he pulled her in for another kiss. His hands tangled in her wet hair, his soft lips reassuring her that this was all they needed, and it almost convinced her it was true. Even though, deep down, a little voice was telling her that he'd never answered the question.

CHAPTER TEN

IF DANIEL COULD just have sat there for ever with Eloise, he'd quite happily have done so. Especially when he was kissing her, all thoughts of the real world fading into insignificance. Being with her held so much promise, a future he'd never deemed possible after he'd lost Anne.

Of course, that in itself burdened him with guilt when he'd sworn there would never be another woman for him—no one with whom he'd want to spend every minute of every day, or who'd ever understand him the way she had. Perhaps because he'd thought he'd never meet that woman who'd tempt him from his self-imposed isolation again. It had seemed improbable to be that fortunate twice in one lifetime.

Now that Eloise appeared to have blown that theory out of the water, it was his decision whether or not he wanted to risk breaking what was left of his heart again if things didn't work out. She wanted a commitment from him, or at the very least a definition of their relationship, but he couldn't give her that. At least, not yet. Opening up his small world to include her in it permanently would mean opening up his heart, being vulnerable again, and he would have to dig deep to find that level of courage before he could commit to that.

'What's that?' Eloise broke the silence that had fallen between them as they finished their tea, and he avoided answering the question.

She anxiously looked around, as though something had spooked her. He hoped they hadn't been spotted by anyone he knew or he would have some explaining to do, pushing him into making a call he really wasn't ready to do.

'I didn't hear anything.' He watched on as Eloise got up and walked away from the small clearing to the leafy bushes nearby.

'Shh. Listen.' She stopped, ears pricked, clearly having heard something he hadn't.

He sat still and quiet, until a chirp finally pierced the silence. It immediately spurred Eloise on in her search, parting the branches, ignoring the jagged brush clawing at her legs in her pursuit.

'Oh, Daniel, he's hurt.'

At the sound of her distress, he got to his feet and went to investigate for himself. She kept the branches parted so he could see what she was looking at: a little starling was hopping around in circles, clearly hurt. Every now and then it gave its wings a flutter but only managed to lift himself partially off the ground.

'It looks as though he's got a broken wing.' Daniel knelt down and cupped his hands gently but firmly around the bird, cradling it as he got to his feet.

'Have we got anything to put him in?'

'The box which had the breakfast pastries in should do.' They made their way back to the blanket and Eloise emptied out the plastic container so they could put the injured bird inside.

'Poor baby,' she soothed, stroking the bird as it pecked at the remaining crumbs in the box. 'Can we help him?'

'I'm sure we can try.' The pleading look she gave him was so full of compassion and hope, there was no way he'd deny the request.

It was clear Eloise was the sort of woman who wore her heart on her sleeve, which made her a vulnerable target for someone who didn't appreciate her. No wonder that the end of her marriage had hurt so much. He knew she'd taken it personally, shouldered the blame and retreated into herself as a result. These were all things he could empathise with when he'd done the same after Anne had died. It was the very reason they were both tiptoeing around the idea of a relationship, even though they were clearly benefitting from being together.

'We can try and make him a splint or something, until it heals.' Eloise pouted, clearly upset on the creature's behalf.

It showed just how nurturing she was and gave Daniel an idea of the kind of loving mother she must be. He had no doubt she paid her daughters the same care and attention she did to everyone else, if not more. She needed somewhere to express those motherly feelings which he was sure hadn't disappeared simply because her children weren't in close proximity. Her daughters didn't know how lucky they were to have her. Not everyone got to grow up in a loving, stable home, which he was sure Eloise had made for her family.

If he was honest, there was a touch of jealousy creeping into his bones at the thought. He would've done anything to have a stable home and family, but it seemed as though Eloise's loved ones didn't know what they'd had. Perhaps if his childhood had been different, if his mother had survived to take care of him, he might've gone on to have a family of his own. As it was, losing his loved ones had traumatised him to the point he hadn't wanted to take the chance of losing anyone else.

Eloise's circumstances had merely cemented that view given, despite a marriage and two daughters, she'd still effectively been left on her own. It wasn't fair on someone who clearly had so much love to give. But even he wouldn't give her the security she needed; he was too afraid himself, of something happening to jeopardise the careful existence he'd established for himself here since Anne had gone.

'We should probably get him back to the clinic with us. I'll X-ray and bandage the wing and phone a rescue centre. They can look after him until he's able to be released.'

Eloise began to pack away their stuff into the bag he'd carried down, but Daniel didn't want to go back to work just yet. It wouldn't be fair to go back to being colleagues, not discussing what had happened and hope it would all work out for the best.

He knew he was being selfish by not being upfront with her about his fears. She needed the same security he did, but in a different way. From their first night together he'd known her fears and problems and had held back his own, afraid to let her see inside to that vulnerable part of him. Now it was time that he was honest with her about why he hadn't been able to man up and put a label on what they had together, what they could have.

'Wait.' He grabbed her hand in his, and she simply stared at it, as though she was afraid this was the last time they'd be able to touch. His heart caught, pained by the fact she knew he'd deny her once they were in company, yet still wanted her in his bed.

'We should go,' she said again, her voice barely a whisper on the wind.

'We will, but first I want to be honest with you about what's happening. How I'm feeling.' He was nauseous at the thought of sharing such personal information, but Eloise deserved to know why he was holding back. Especially when it wasn't her fault.

She sat back, listening, waiting for him to open his heart. Even their little one-winged patient had stopped chirping, giving him the floor to speak without interruption. All he had to do was find the courage to use his voice.

'I like being with you,' he started.

'Thank goodness for that.' Eloise attempted to lighten the sudden tension between them and he appreciated that she was trying to make this easier for him.

'You have to understand that growing up in

care, constantly moving around foster homes and living with different people, wasn't easy. It was hard for me to feel secure, or to get close to people, because I knew I'd inevitably have to move again. I'd already lost my mother, didn't know my father and it was too hard to keep making friends or getting close to a family, only to move on again. So I learned to keep an emotional distance, preventing my heart from taking another battering.

'Then I met Anne… Up until then, my relationships had been short-term, casual, and work was the only thing I fully committed to. She showed me that we wanted the same things, but we could still have a good time, enjoy one another's company. Anne showed me how not to be afraid to love again. Then she died.'

'And you hid yourself away from the world again.'

Eloise got it. She seemed to understand him in a way no one else did.

'It seems safer that way. I hadn't counted on meeting you. On getting close.'

'Neither had I. I didn't think I'd ever get that lucky.' Her compliment warmed his insides even more than the flask of tea. Yet he didn't want her to think that he was the answer to all her problems. There was a long way to go for both of them.

'The thing is…it's a big step for me to have anyone in my life. It's going to take a while to get used to.'

'I can wait. It's not like I'm going anywhere soon.'

'I just… I need to process the fact that I'm moving on. That I *want* to move on. Until then, I'd like to carry on the way we are—getting to know one another, spending time together, making love…'

Even saying it, thinking about it, made him want her all over again. If it wasn't for the fact they had to get to work, or that someone might see them, he'd take her right this minute. As tempting as outdoor sex was, they had reputations and jobs to protect, and were supposedly mature enough to keep their libidos in check until they had somewhere private to go. It might make it even hotter when they would have to hold back until after work.

'I think we can manage that.' Eloise leaned over and gave him a sweet peck on the lips, which he hoped was something they'd get to expand on later.

Everything he had with Eloise was something to look forward to; sharing his working day, having dinner together, even walking the dog, were all tasks much improved by having her as a partner. In their own way they were becoming a little family, with Lucky and their new little patient to take care of together. It was something he'd always been too afraid to want. All he had to do now was let go of that damaged foster child inside so he could get on with this new life being offered to him.

'Daniel? What are you doing here? I told you I'm out of action for the foreseeable future.' Eloise rubbed her eyes and pulled her dressing gown tighter around her body as the cold air filtered in from the open door.

She'd thought something was wrong when her doorbell had rung at this hour of the morning, but Daniel was standing on her doorstep with Lucky, both looking happy to see her.

'That doesn't mean we have to miss breakfast. It was hard enough not waking up to you this morning. For future reference, I'm happy to just cuddle, as long as that means you'll stay over.' He pushed past her into the house and in the kitchen began unpacking the bag he was carrying, with a loyal Lucky trotting in behind him.

'Well, come on in,' she said, unbothered by the interruption to her lie-in.

They'd got into something of a routine before work: waking up, going for a swim then having breakfast. Of course, the best part of all of that for her was sitting having tea with him, but she was getting used to the ice-cold wake-up call too.

It was difficult, not touching each other at work, but they'd been careful not to let their 'relationship' spill over into the work environment. As far as she was aware, they'd managed to keep it secret from their colleagues, but she looked forward to closing time. Then she'd slip into Daniel's house for dinner, and more often than not she'd stay the night.

Even though she'd prefer to have more of a commitment, to put her mind at ease that he wasn't going to decide he didn't want anything more than a casual arrangement, she was happy enough with the situation for now. It was more than she'd ever expected to have when she'd moved here.

The only fly in the ointment at present was her unreliable hormones, which had sprung some breakthrough bleeding on her. She wasn't due her period for another week, but her bedroom adventures with Daniel had been curtailed for now, along with the swimming. They seemed to be on the same page, though, with being together seeming more important than the physical aspect of their evenings. It was that intimacy she missed.

'Do you want proper cups or the usual?' He waved the little metallic mugs she'd come to know and love, since it was a symbol of their early morning quality time together, rain or shine.

'There's no point in breaking the habit. It almost tastes better out of those.' She stood by and let him fix their usual selection of pastries and fruit, along with their tea. He looked at home in her kitchen, and she loved that he'd even thought to do this for her.

Her problems had been nothing but an inconvenience to Sam; how she was feeling had been immaterial. He'd only been concerned with how it impacted on his life. Selfish—a word that could never be used to describe Daniel. She saw the way he interacted with the sick and injured animals at work, and the owners, who sometimes needed a little more careful handling. He gave a lot, and never expected anything in return. That was something she wasn't used to.

'It's nice to do this in the warmth for once, don't you think?' Daniel handed her a cup and carried their indoor picnic into the living room.

'Do you know what would be even nicer?'

she asked, taking a bite of a sugar-glazed donut he must have bought especially, knowing what a sweet tooth she had.

'What's that?' Daniel helped himself to a nectarine, the juice dribbling down his chin as he bit into it.

Everything about this man was a turn-on, which in itself was like getting blood from a stone. Before him, she'd thought her body had given up on the idea of being with anyone again. Now she knew differently...though there was only one man she wanted to be with, who made her feel this way.

Regardless that neither of them wanted to label their relationship, both afraid of their feelings and scarred by the past, she knew she was falling for him. She'd jumped right in at the deep end, and was struggling to keep her head above water, because she knew already that if he decided to end things she would be devastated.

'Breakfast in bed; maybe on a Sunday morning, when we don't have to get up for work.' She could picture it, them cosied up together, spending the whole day in bed, making love and snacking on pastries. *Heaven.*

'I'm sure that can be easily arranged when you're feeling better. If you want to come over tonight, I'm making spaghetti. I've also got chocolate and a hot-water bottle if you want to cuddle up on the sofa and watch a soppy film.'

Eloise watched him through suspicious eyes. 'Have you been typing "perfect man" into a search engine, trying to impress me?'

He was saying all the right things, offering comfort food and emotional support. There had to be a catch somewhere.

'Am I being too OTT? Sorry. I just felt as though I never did enough for Anne when she was going through this and I want to be there for you.'

Even the words, without the gesture, were enough to bring her to tears, just knowing he wanted to help. He never made her feel like a burden, or an inconvenience, despite her crashing into his life and upending his routine.

'I'm sure Anne was grateful to you just for being there. I know I am. You don't have to go to any trouble for me. Although, I'd love some comfort food…and chocolate. I'll take you instead of the hot-water bottle, and there's no need for a soppy movie. I'm a bit too cynical for those these days. I'd settle for a thriller.'

She didn't care what they would watch; it would just be nice to cuddle up with him, with no expectation of pretending that she was up for anything else. There was no telling where their new arrangement was going to lead, but Eloise knew she wanted it to last.

Her phone rang then, the outside world breaking into their morning ritual. When she saw her eldest daughter Dawn's name on the screen, her heart became more full than it had in ages. Those lonely days rattling around the house on her own with nothing to look forward to, no one to talk to, seemed a lifetime away now. Since coming here, she had someone to be with, to look forward to a future with, and she knew being happier in herself would mean being a better mother. Moving here was the best thing she'd done in years and she hoped it would stay that way.

'It's my daughter,' Eloise told him as she grabbed her phone. 'Do you mind if I take this?'

'Of course not.'

She didn't want to be rude by taking the call, but neither did she want to ignore it. As excited as Eloise was to hear from Dawn, she worried that there might be something wrong.

'Hi, honey. Is everything okay?' She paced across the living room floor, that worry clutching at her stomach until she was assured that her daughter was all right.

'Hi, Mum. Everything's fine. I just wanted

to call you with some news. Curtis and I are having a baby.'

'What?' That tension lifted, her spirits soaring with the happy news and her daughter's obvious joy at becoming a mother herself. She just wanted to make sure she hadn't imagined it.

'I'm pregnant. I wanted to wait until the third-month scan to make sure everything's okay with the baby.'

'And is it?'

'Yes. Everything's great. We're over the moon.'

'I'm so happy for you. That's wonderful news, so exciting for everyone. I'm sure your sister will be delighted to find out she's going to be an auntie.'

'And you're going to be a granny. Or would you prefer "Nanny"? Maybe "Glam-ma"?' she teased.

'Granny's fine. I'm not bothered about titles. I'm just over the moon that you're going to have a little one of your own.' She turned to grin at Daniel to let him in on the happy news too. He gave her a thumbs-up, and for a brief moment she pictured babysitting her grandchild with him.

Then the pretty picture dissipated when she remembered that her daughter lived in another country and she'd be lucky even to get a cuddle with the new member of the family. As much as she was enjoying her new life here, she was still mourning her old one. Now she'd have even more reason to miss her daughters and her role in their lives. Even Daniel wasn't going to fill that void in her heart that her family had left, and it was only going to get bigger by the day, knowing there would now be a baby for her to miss too.

'I'm going to be a mum,' Dawn whispered, as though she couldn't believe it was true.

Emotion choked Eloise now; she was thrilled for her, but sad for herself that she wasn't going to be a part of that journey with her. If she was lucky, she'd get to be an occasional visitor into their lives—something that wasn't currently working out too well for her.

'You're going to be wonderful.' Her voice cracked, the effort of holding back finally becoming too much. She turned away from Daniel so he wouldn't see her tears, even though he could probably hear them.

'Actually, Mum, it's got me thinking… I want you to be part of this. To be in our lives. I don't want my baby to grow up not knowing you. You'd make such a wonderful grandmother.'

'But I don't know how that would work.' It was breaking her heart already, knowing that she wasn't going to see this baby grow up and be part of all of those firsts that she'd gone through with her own children.

Her ex-husband had always been the main breadwinner and she'd taken care of things at home. That had meant being the more involved parent, attending school meetings and plays, arranging play dates and making sure big occasions such as birthdays and Christmas were special. The chance to do all of that again, or at least be included in it, was something she'd thought she'd never get to have. Now it was almost within her reach again, it was torture that only distance would keep her from it.

Dawn cleared her throat. 'Well, we've been talking it over, and you know we have a huge house here? I know you're on your own over there and I thought maybe, you know, you might want to move in with us. You could help me with child care when I go back to work, or just be there. I miss you, Mum.'

'I miss you too, sweetheart.' If she'd had this offer a couple of weeks earlier, Eloise wouldn't have thought twice about taking Dawn up on the idea. Now, however, she'd set up a new life for herself. She had someone here she cared about, a job, a house and a future of her own.

It was a pity there wasn't a way for her to have it all.

'Anyway, you have plenty of time to think it over. I better go call Dad and share the news.'

Eloise could only imagine how that news was going to go down with Sam when he was so caught up with reliving his youth. Becoming a grandad certainly wouldn't be such an exciting prospect for him, she was sure. It was very telling that he wasn't being invited to help raise the new addition to the family.

'Okay, sweetheart. Congratulations again, and I'll definitely think the offer over.'

'I hope you decide to come. I miss you. Bye, Mum.'

'Talk to you later. Bye.'

She ended the call and flopped down into a chair, emotionally wiped out by the exchange.

'Good news, I take it? Congratulations.' Daniel raised his cup of tea to her.

'Thanks. It's a lot to take in. I'm too young to be a granny,' she protested with a laugh, even though it really didn't bother her at all.

'When's the baby due?'

'You know, I didn't even ask the exact date, but she's three months gone. She's asked me if I would like to move out there with them and be more of a hands-on grandmother.'

'Oh? And that…that's something you'd want to do?' Despite Daniel's carefully worded question, she understood the meaning behind it. He wanted to know if she was going to leave him.

'Yes and no. I have a life here I'm not ready to abandon. But it's something I'm going to have to at least consider.'

'Of course.'

After he'd opened up to her about his past, and why he didn't want to get close to anyone, Eloise understood why he'd be concerned about this new development.

Eloise wished she didn't have to make a decision between him and her family at all, but at least she had a few months to think about it. To see how things went with Daniel and her, and if he'd prove serious competition for her new grandchild when it came to sharing her life and her heart.

CHAPTER ELEVEN

'IT'S BEEN QUITE a day, hasn't it?' Eloise finished wiping down the examination table, then took a handkerchief and mopped Daniel's brow.

He forced a laugh, glad that they'd been busy today so it hadn't left them a lot of time to talk. After the phone call that morning, he'd been somewhat at a loss for words. Eloise hearing from her daughter, and her otherwise happy news, had left him feeling on the outside of her life and it made him uncomfortable.

Things were fine when they were in their little bubble of two, where none of their real worries were allowed to enter. That contact from her family changed everything. Though he was glad for her sake that someone other than he could finally see her worth, it was forcing them to take stock of their relationship—something he'd been shying away from with good reason it seemed.

This was everything that he'd been afraid of.

The second he'd opened his heart, fate had conspired to take her away from him…unless he was honest about his feelings for her. He knew he'd fallen hard, and that was why he was so afraid of committing. But if he wasn't up front about how much she meant to him, how much he wanted her in his life, she mightn't think there was anything worth staying here for.

He resolved to have an honest conversation with her over dinner tonight. Then at least she'd have all the facts at hand when she made her decision.

Just as they turned off the lights in the surgery, getting ready for the best part of his day when they were alone in his place, someone started hammering on the front door.

'Can someone help? Please.' The woman on the doorstep looked desperate, clutching the hand of a toddler and cradling something in her other hand.

'I guess the day isn't over just yet.' Daniel wouldn't turn anyone away and immediately unlocked the door to admit one more patient.

'Come on through.' Eloise turned the lights back on and led the latecomers through to the exam room she'd just cleaned down.

'He's just started fitting. I don't know what's

wrong with him.' The woman set a rabbit and the blanket it was wrapped in down on the table.

The little boy with her was obviously upset at witnessing his pet's distress, and Daniel couldn't be sure at this stage he could even save the rabbit.

'Hey, sweetheart. What's your bunny's name?' Eloise, who was clearly on the same page, knelt down to speak to the child, distracting him from what was going on.

'Angus.'

'That's a lovely name. Did you call him that?'

The boy nodded.

'I'm Eloise, and the man taking care of your rabbit is Daniel. What's your name?'

He looked at his mum for confirmation it was okay for him to share that information with a stranger. When she gave him the go-ahead, he muttered a shy, 'Frankie.'

'Well, Frankie, why don't we let Daniel and your mum talk in here and we'll go and find something fun to do?' Eloise took the boy's hand and turned to Daniel, mouthing, 'Is that okay?'

He waved her away, keen to get the child out as soon as possible, knowing that there was probably little he could do for the animal except give it pain relief and hope the seizures stopped soon.

The sound of Eloise's voice carried down the corridor as she engaged with the little boy, and his excited response as she took him into the waiting room. Daniel had seen her on occasion, helping the kids colour in when they were waiting for news on their beloved pets, or holding babies for anxious parents trying to juggle animals and toddlers. It was obvious she was born to mother and he could only imagine how happy her family life had made her before everyone had gone their separate ways. It was probably as much a vocation for her as her job, if not more.

He supposed her role here was scant consolation for the one she'd lost, as was he. Going swimming, watching TV and sleeping over wasn't much to offer in comparison to her having that family life again. It wouldn't be fair to keep her here, pretending that he could ever fill that void in her life where her children, and now her grandchildren, had a right to be. It was tempting to beg her to stay so he didn't lose her, but it would also be selfish.

He couldn't promise her any of the things she clearly needed in her life, like children or family. Neither could he be sure that whatever this was would last, or make it worth the heartbreak for either of them. If he couldn't completely open up to her, it would be a betrayal to them both. As far as he could see, letting this thing between them go on any longer would simply end in pain, and they'd both had enough of that to last lifetimes.

At least by letting her go now, on his terms, he'd save himself some of that heartbreak just waiting round the corner when she decided he hadn't been worth the sacrifice after all.

One of them deserved to be happy, and he could go back to the way his life had been before Eloise had made him think he could have something more. Now he just had to tell her it was over and she wouldn't have to choose between a couple of strays and her real family, who still needed her.

'Bless him; little Frankie wanted to make a "get well soon" card for his bunny.' Eloise barely made it into Daniel's house before collapsing onto the sofa. It had been a physical and emotionally draining day. She was glad he wasn't expecting anything more than dinner and a cuddle.

Daniel winced. 'I'm not sure that's going to happen if the rabbit doesn't stop fitting or start eating soon. I've sedated him and he's been given fluids. I'll check on him again after dinner, but given his age I don't think he's going to make it. I explained the situation to the mother so I think she's going to try and break the news to her little boy so it doesn't come as such a shock.'

'Aww, that's sad, but children are resilient. When Alison's hamster, Biscuit, died she was sad until we took her out to get another one—then Biscuit Mark Two became the best thing since sliced bread. It's important for them to learn about death and grief. Although, I hope when I go they'll mourn me long after the next Mrs Carter comes on the scene.'

Losing a pet was the hardest, and the worst part of being both an owner and working at the clinic. Some things were simply out of their control, and Eloise was definitely happier when she had some power over what was happening, although today's events were testing that theory.

She had a big decision to make about her future and it was sure to cause more than a few sleepless nights. Her family had always come first, but that was how she'd ended up alone when they'd all moved on, with no life of her own. It had taken her time, perseverance and Daniel's help to get where she was now. She didn't want to just abandon the life she'd made here for herself.

Yet, the prospect of being part of a family again was exciting, and everything she'd wanted. If only there was a way to have it all, she'd be one very lucky woman. But that wasn't the way life worked out for her. Something would have to give, and it was going to be painful, whatever happened.

No doubt Daniel was thinking the same, as he'd been quieter than usual at work, and even during dinner. Even now, instead of the promised snuggling in front of the TV, they were sitting at opposite ends of the sofa. It was as though by distancing themselves from one another they could avoid the subject she knew had to be addressed sooner or later.

'I'm not sure if I want to be a full-time nanny to my own grandchild.' She hadn't meant to spit it out like that, but she'd been thinking about it all day, and he was the only person she could talk to about it.

'Why not?' He stopped stroking Lucky, who was lying on the floor at his feet, so he could turn his attention to her instead.

'I mean, of course I want to spend time with him, or her, and any other future grandchildren.

I just don't know if that's all I want. I have a life here now.'

Deep down, she was hoping Daniel was going to declare his undying love for her and beg her to stay, taking the decision out of her hands. Because she knew where she wanted to be…and that was right here.

'Don't pin all your hopes on me, Eloise.'

He fixed her with a dark stare that she hadn't seen from him before. It chilled her, freezing the blood in her veins that had been pumping with excitement at the prospect of a future with him until now.

'Don't you want me to stay?' She almost couldn't get the words out, she was so aghast. With the way things had been between them, she hadn't really considered that. Yes, she knew they'd have some challenges to work through when they were both carrying so much baggage from the past, but she'd thought they were at least on the same page as far as their relationship went. That they wanted to be together.

As Daniel leaned forward, looking down at his feet instead of meeting her eye, she realised he thought differently.

'It's not about me, or at least it shouldn't be. You know I'm not ready to commit to anything, I've been clear about that.'

'I knew you had concerns about getting hurt—not that you didn't *want* something more between us.' That changed everything. He was right, in that she wouldn't give up the chance to be with her family and have a life including them if all that remained here was an empty house and only herself for company. She'd had that for too long and she needed more to fulfil her.

Except, Eloise thought that she'd found more for herself here: Daniel. She didn't want to pin everything on him, but he'd helped her find herself again. It wouldn't be inconceivable to want that to continue. Though she should have learned her lesson on relying on others to give her existence meaning. She was always going to be left scrabbling to find a life of her own when they didn't need her any more.

'I said I wanted to carry on with what we were doing. If you stay on account of me, instead of going to be with your family, you're asking something of me that I'm not ready to give.'

Daniel shrugged, proving he wasn't as bothered as she was about the whole situation. It was clear cut for him, and perhaps it would be easier if she was no longer in the picture at all. She'd been a fool again.

'And what would I do here in the meantime? It will take a while to sort things out and the baby isn't even due for another six months.'

Now she had no other option but to leave if Daniel didn't feel for her what she did for him. Her feelings were too deep to stick around and see him every day, knowing that he couldn't be hers. Besides, she'd spent enough of her life putting other people's needs and wants before her own, and Daniel had made her see she was worthy of someone's love. If it was never going to be him, there was no point staying and mooning after him, fighting her feelings every day just to keep other people happy.

She'd have to go. That would mean selling up, moving or storing all of her belongings and working out the logistics of moving to another country. They were things she hoped she could sort out sooner rather than later, because she didn't think she could stand months of being around him and being reminded of everything she'd lost. That if he'd been brave enough, or loved her enough, they could've had a future.

Perhaps it was simply because *she* wasn't enough for him. All those thoughts she'd had, that he'd support her through menopause and anything else, had been apparently no more than wishful thinking. No doubt if she'd been one of those sexy, slim, elegant women approaching her fifties she might've had a shot. She'd been fooling herself by thinking otherwise. All she'd been was convenient…until now.

'I told you your job would be safe no matter what happened between us. It'll take me a while to find a replacement anyway.' He was so matter of fact about the end of their relationship, such as it was, she wondered why she'd invested so much in it.

Now he'd taken a step beyond his mourning, at least into a physical arrangement, he might eventually move on to a proper relationship some day. Apparently that wouldn't be with her and it made her think that he wouldn't look for a replacement for just her role in the clinic.

As for her, it would be a while before she put herself out there again. She supposed she should be thankful she'd had one last fling before she'd been completely written off. At least if she moved out to be with her daughter she wouldn't find herself on the scrapheap altogether.

Eloise stared at him, at a loss for words, because those nights together, not to mention their mornings, didn't seem to mean anything to him when it had been everything to her. She knew that companionship, the reason to get up in the mornings and the passion she'd thought had long gone were all things she wouldn't have with anyone else when it had taken her this long to find them.

'So, what was this tonight—a last supper?' She'd been looking forward to everything; now it just seemed like a cruel joke, with her pasta dinner now weighing heavily in her stomach.

'I made you a promise…'

The bitter, 'Ha!' that escaped her lips wasn't planned, but appropriate. She supposed technically he hadn't made her a promise where their relationship was concerned, but it had been implied—in her mind, at least.

Somehow this felt like an even bigger betrayal than her husband leaving her after thirty years of marriage. Most likely, because she'd opened up to Daniel more than she ever had to Sam. It showed the lack of communication they'd had, that she hadn't been able to tell him how she was feeling, or vice versa, before it had been too late. Daniel had never said, or done, any of the hurtful things to her that her husband had at the end of their relationship, but this was still painful, because his strength of feeling for her wasn't enough for him to fight for her, even to ask her to stay.

That was enough to make the tears well up

in her eyes, and she knew she had to leave before she made a scene. She could do her weeping and wailing at home, in private, where there would be no one to see or hear her because she was all alone. And she would have to get it out of her system tonight. After all, she would be expected to go to work in the morning as though nothing had happened. As though her heart hadn't just been freshly ripped from her chest.

'I suppose there's no point in drawing this out, in that case. I'll see you at work tomorrow.'

Eloise grabbed her things and walked out without a backward glance. She didn't give him a chance to talk her round. She'd be too weak to resist if he suggested that they carry on until it was time for her to go, and that would only make it even harder for her to leave.

As she got into her car, tears now blurring her vision, it occurred to her that he hadn't even tried.

CHAPTER TWELVE

'I'm so sorry I'm late.' Eloise bustled into the clinic, aware that she looked a mess. There'd been no time to do her make-up or do anything more than run a brush through her hair by the time she woke up. Daniel would probably realise he'd had a lucky escape when he saw her.

She'd spent most of the night crying, eating and replaying every second they'd spent together since she'd moved here. Wondering how she'd got it so wrong, believing they'd had something special when it clearly meant nothing to him. Perhaps she'd just been so desperate for some affection and attention, she'd read more into it than sex with her boss. Perhaps it was a cliché, not some grand love affair, after all.

'I'm just glad you're here.' Brooke handed her some paperwork before she'd even had time to take off her coat.

It had been tempting to phone in sick rather

than face Daniel this morning, but she hadn't wanted to let down her colleagues, who were clearly under enough pressure this morning with a full waiting room. Her subconscious had probably decided for her that a lie-in was called for in order to avoid him, but guilt had got the better of her when she had finally woken up. Now she had to face the man who'd kept her awake with crying over him.

She took a deep breath as she opened the door to the examination room, only to find a complete stranger in a white coat injecting a Pomeranian.

'Sorry,' she said, and closed the door again.

When she checked the other room in case Daniel had moved for some reason, she found Debbie working there instead.

'Where's Daniel?' she asked Brooke.

'Oh, he's taken a leave of absence.'

'Pardon?' She'd been working herself up to come here and he'd taken the easy way out? He really wasn't the man she'd thought he was.

'I know.' Brooke leaned forward with a conspiratorial whisper. 'I've never known him to go on holiday or even take a sick day. Apparently he phoned Debbie at an ungodly hour this morning telling her he'd got cover and would be off indefinitely.'

'He didn't say why, or where, he was going?'

Brooke shrugged. 'That's all I was told. I would've thought if anyone would know it would be you.'

She spun round, back to her computer, dropping the bombshell that they hadn't managed to keep anything secret from their colleagues after all. The only thing more humiliating than that would be having to tell them that he was too embarrassed even to be in the same building as her. Although, they'd probably worked that out for themselves by now.

Daniel skimmed a stone across the loch, watching the ripples as it bounced, causing a disturbance in the calm water before disappearing altogether. Much like Eloise, who'd burst into his quiet life, forced him out of his comfort zone and caused ripples that were going to affect him long after she'd left the country. Yet he didn't regret a moment with her.

Lucky came and sat beside him at the edge of the loch, tail wagging, panting and as loyal as ever.

'You wouldn't be this happy if you knew that it's just me you're going to be stuck with from now on,' he told the oblivious dog.

Daniel supposed at least he would have some

company once Eloise had gone to live with her family. Even if he could never hope a stray mutt could give him the companionship or dreams for a better future he knew he would've had with her. He hoped that by letting her go now she'd have a more fulfilling life with her family rather than just plodding along with him. She deserved more than he had to give.

That didn't mean he wasn't in pain, feeling as though he was mourning a lost love all over again. It would probably seem to Eloise that he'd taken the cowardly way out by getting cover in at work, but the truth was that he didn't think he'd be able to hold it together, seeing her at work, knowing that she was going to leave any day. At least this way he had some control. That was what he was trying to convince himself.

He couldn't even bear to be in his own house, his own bed, without her. Since Anne had died, he'd convinced himself he could go it alone. He'd had his love and, now it had gone, he simply had to get on with his life, such as it was. Eloise had changed that way of thinking, had shown him a different world with her in it, but he'd lost her the moment her daughter had called.

Now he had to try and get back to life the

way it had been before Eloise had disrupted his peace of mind. So he'd rented one of the cabins at the farthest end of the loch from the practice for a few days. Usually it was fishermen or couples on a romantic break who stayed here, away from civilisation, but it was just the dog and him.

He didn't know how long it would take for him to get his head straight before he went back to work and faced Eloise. She wasn't happy with him, or the way he'd ended things, but he hoped that would make the decision to leave easier for her. One day she'd see that and forgive him. The best thing he could probably do for both of them was to stay here, away from the memories, until she left—though he knew that wasn't practical. A couple of days' distancing himself would have to suffice for now.

The sound of splashing and laughter sounded nearby and, perhaps bored with only Daniel's company, Lucky took off to find whoever was nearby. He was probably hoping it was Eloise, come to rescue him again. Daniel jogged along the small strip of shore at the edge of the water, calling him. Apparently they still needed to work on their recall training.

'Lucky, get back here.' Following the excited

barks, he found the escapee mesmerised by the sight of a couple swimming in the loch.

'Sorry. I didn't mean to disturb you. He just ran off.' He called to the elderly pair watching bemusedly as he tried to get Lucky back on his lead.

'That's all right. We're just getting out now.' The man, who Daniel guessed to be in his late seventies, began to stride out, grabbed up hooded robes from the shore and handed one to his wife.

'The cup of tea is the best part. Would you like one?' The woman offered up her flask in one hand and a box of cupcakes in the other.

Daniel smiled. 'That's very kind of you, but I didn't mean to intrude.'

The scene reminded him of the mornings he and Eloise had spent doing the same thing. Not the most thrilling adventure of all time to some people, but it had come to mean so much to him. So much, in fact, that he hadn't been able to go swimming without her since.

'Not at all. We're so used to just seeing each other, it's nice to see a different face for once.' She nudged him with the box of goodies and he decided it would be rude to refuse a second time.

'Do you live near here?' He didn't recognise

their faces, although that didn't mean much when he didn't socialise a lot outside of work. Unless they were pet owners, he wasn't likely to have met them before even if they only lived down the road.

'Glasgow. We're just staying in one of the cabins for a couple of nights. It's so peaceful here.' She glanced around the vast wooded area around them, and it reminded Daniel of Eloise's reaction when she'd first arrived.

'It's definitely a change of pace.' He had hoped that this space on his own would help him reset, but it no longer held quite the same appeal.

'Don't get me wrong, I wouldn't like to be here on my own, but Matthew is my rock. Without him it feels like I'm missing a limb.' The woman's words struck him so hard, Daniel felt as though he'd been winded.

'Well, I hope you enjoy your break together. I should get this one back for his dinner, and thanks for the cupcake.' Daniel took Lucky and his sweet treat back to his own cabin, with the stranger's comment ringing in his ears.

When Anne had died, he'd had to adapt to life alone, but Eloise had opened the world up to him again. Losing her, and the possibilities she brought to his life, did make him feel as though part of him was missing: his heart.

The difference between losing Anne and losing Eloise was that his current state was his choice. As if he'd willingly, and bizarrely, decided just to chop off a limb and throw it away—something he'd apparently rather do than simply face up to his feelings and take a chance on love again. This lonely existence he faced again seemed scant consolation when she'd be gone for ever.

He'd thought he was content living and working here, but having her in his life had showed him what real happiness felt like. If he let her go without even trying to make a relationship work, then he really would be the coward she likely thought him now.

That was, if she even wanted him. He couldn't make her choose between her family and him, but the prospect of being without her now seemed more bleak than a future here with his heart still intact—never taking that risk.

To win her back, he was going to have to prove just how much he was willing to commit to her.

'Snookie McDaniels, please.' Usually calling out some of the more amusing pet names made a busy day a little bit brighter, but Eloise hadn't found much to smile about lately.

Without Daniel, this place wasn't somewhere she'd looked forward to coming to any more. Though she was still waking up at six every morning, lying awake, missing their swimming and outdoor breakfasts. She supposed she'd have to get used to it. No one seemed to know when Daniel was coming back, and at this point she wouldn't be surprised if he waited until she'd gone. Her exciting new start appeared to have come to a prematurely sad end.

The family with Snookie the sick tortoise came through to the new vet, who was nice enough, but Eloise couldn't bring herself to move past small talk with him. She was missing Daniel too much. Only time would tell if distance would ease that pain in her heart where he'd taken up residence.

The phone in her pocket vibrated with an incoming call: Dawn. Eloise declined the call and turned her phone off. She'd told her daughter that she was going to move out, and ever since had been plagued with calls about getting organised. Understandable, she supposed, except once she put her house on the market it would make it all real. It really would be over between Daniel and her, and part of her still hopelessly wished she could have it all: a life here with Daniel, her job and still seeing her children and grandchild.

'Eloise, can I talk to you next door?' As though she'd conjured him with thought alone, Daniel came striding in through the clinic door and straight to her.

'What? I'm working.' Her mind was filled with a million questions, but her immediate thought was that he looked good with a few days' stubble.

'I need to speak to you.' He grabbed her arm and there was a desperation in his eyes she couldn't ignore.

'Can you...?' She turned to Brooke, who was watching their interplay with fascination.

'I'll tell him you got called away to an emergency,' she said with a smile.

'Thanks.' Eloise's heart was thumping against her rib cage, her stomach like a whirlpool as she followed Daniel, wondering what on earth was so important.

Lucky greeted her at the door with an enthusiastic lick and she bent down to hug him.

'I've missed you.' Words she wanted to say to Daniel but knew she couldn't.

'We missed you too,' Daniel told her, easing some of that pain in her chest.

'Where did you go?' She tried to keep the pain out of her voice, but it made her sound so small.

'I just needed some space to think. Sorry.'

'And…and what conclusion did you come to?' She held her breath, waiting, hoping that, since ending their relationship hadn't been as easy for him as she'd thought, he'd had some regret.

Daniel took her hands and pulled her up from her crouched position on the floor. 'That I don't want to lose you, Eloise.'

It was everything she wanted to hear, but it didn't solve any problems other than soothing her ego. She still had to make a decision about whether to stay here and take a chance on someone who'd just denied her, or be part of her family's lives again.

'I thought you weren't that bothered. In fact, I think you told me to go.'

He flinched, as though she'd just punched him. 'I thought I was doing the right thing by you. And I was afraid I was going to lose you anyway, so I thought…'

'That you'd just speed things along.'

'Something like that.' He gave her a cute smile that made him look like a mischievous little boy who'd been caught after breaking a window with his football.

'So where do we go from here? You haven't even told me how you feel about me. I mean, I need to know that before I go making any life changing decisions...' Before she could finish, Daniel took her in his arms and kissed her hard on the lips.

'I love you, Eloise. I was afraid to admit it until now, because that means leaving myself open to getting hurt again if you leave.'

All things he'd told her before, but she hadn't realised they related to her until now. It was no wonder he'd got spooked with the possibility of her moving to another country. But, by saying those three words, he'd complicated everything even more for her. Now there was a reason to stay: the future with Daniel she'd been hoping for might actually be within her reach. Except, she'd already told her daughter that she would move to be with her.

'I've told Dawn that I'm going to go and live with her.'

'Is that what you really want?' He wasn't playing fair with her. She wanted to be with him, but he wasn't guaranteeing her for ever, and anything less than that was a risk. At least Dawn was offering love and support she knew she could count on, even if it was of an altogether different kind.

'I want everything. I want to be with you, and my family, but that isn't possible.'

'And I want to be with you.'

'I don't doubt that, Daniel, at least for now, but what if you change your mind again? You can't just disappear and not tell me what's going on in your head. You have to talk to me so we can work through any problems together. That's what people in a relationship do.'

She was putting that out there. She wanted a relationship and everything that came with it. If that wasn't what he wanted too, then they'd be doomed from the outset, and she wasn't going to go through the pain of another break-up if she could help it.

'I know. I'm sorry. I guess I just have to get used to being part of a couple again.' He gave her that half-smile that made her want to forgive him anything.

'You really want to give us a chance?' She was afraid to ask, because his answer was going to change all the plans she'd been making for her future.

'Yes. I know I was an idiot but I was afraid that you were going to leave me eventually and break my heart anyway. I don't want to lose you, Eloise. I love you.'

He was being honest with her, opening up about how he felt and why he'd acted the way he had. It was all she could ask from him. Now it was down to her to decide what she wanted to do about this new revelation. Her heart told her that Daniel was worth taking a chance on.

'Maybe that's a risk we both have to take if we want to be together. I love you too, Daniel. We'll make this work.'

'I've done a lot of thinking over these past few days, and I would rather be with you anywhere in the world than here on my own. I could move over there with you, if you wanted me to.'

Daniel's revelation that he would give up everything that he'd worked so hard for here to go with her was the biggest commitment he could make to her, but she could never ask him to do that. He'd been brave, and now it was her turn.

'I wouldn't ask that of you, Daniel. All I wanted was to know that you felt the same way about me that I do about you. If there's a chance that we can be together, keep on working together, swimming, sharing a bed, I'm never going to give that up.'

'What about your daughter and your grandchild? I can't ask you to just forget about them.'

'That's never going to happen. I can visit and video-call, just like I have been doing. I'm still going to be in their lives. You will be too, hopefully.'

'I think I'd like that. To be part of a family.' He smiled, and Eloise saw the scarred little boy finally realise that he was loved and wanted.

It was exactly how he made her feel too. And neither of them was going anywhere without the other any time soon. They'd found their purpose, and their future, in each other.

EPILOGUE

One year later

'DO YOU THINK there's going to be enough room for them all? Maybe they should sleep in our room.' Eloise was trying to think of everything that Dawn and her little family were going to need to be comfortable for their stay.

'They're going to be fine. Happy just to be here with you.' Daniel put his hands on her shoulders and talked her down from spiralling into a great ball of anxiety.

'I just want everything to be right.' Although she'd been lucky enough to fly out to Canberra with Daniel to see baby Gabby just after her birth, meeting up with Alison out there too, she hadn't seen them in person since. She knew she'd made the right decision in staying here with Daniel, but it didn't mean she didn't still miss being with her family.

'You've gone to a lot of trouble, making the

place lovely for them. Stop worrying.' He shut her up the way he knew how, with a kiss.

Since finally facing their fears and committing to one another, they'd gone all in. Daniel had moved into her place, keen for a completely new start away from the marital home he'd shared with Anne. Debbie was renting it now, so everyone was happy with the arrangement.

Life had been good. They spent every day together, working and winding down at home afterwards, which usually ended in some passionate love-making. The mornings were good too, and she even looked forward to the cold dip as much as the outdoor breakfast they shared.

She was just worried something was going to happen to spoil it, even though she knew her daughters were both fond of Daniel and were happy she'd found someone who appreciated and loved her. Alison had even talked about doing some house hunting when they were over. There was a possibility her husband could get a work transfer, and she missed Eloise as much as Eloise missed her daughter and granddaughter. So she had her fingers crossed that she could have everything after all.

'Do you think Lucky should stay outside? I wouldn't want him to upset the baby.'

'Eloise, you know he's great around people. Stop panicking. Everything's going to be okay.'

He was right. Lucky was quite the celebrity at the clinic now, happy to lie quietly at Reception, or entertain the children who came in and liked to make a fuss of him.

'I don't know how you put up with me sometimes.' She wrapped her arms around his waist and laid her head against his chest—her favourite place in the world to be, where she felt safe and loved.

'Because I love you.' He kissed the top of her head and hugged her closer.

Eloise had no doubts on that score. He'd been with her through everything, including the not so pleasant side effects of peri-menopause. He was always there with a hot water bottle, or a fan, or a cup of tea. She didn't know how she'd got so lucky.

'I love you too,' she mumbled into his chest.

'Hold that thought.' Suddenly, he pushed her away and walked out of the room, leaving her wondering what she'd done to send him away.

Thankfully he came back not long after… though she hadn't expected him to drop to one knee.

'I was going to wait until your family were here to celebrate, but I think this is the perfect time. I just hope I can get up off this floor again.'

He was joking around, but Eloise's heart was in her mouth, waiting for him to get to the point.

'Perfect time for what?'

'To ask you to marry me. Eloise Carter, would you do me the honour of becoming my wife?' He opened a box to show her a beautiful diamond ring inside and she thought her heart would burst with happiness.

'Yes. I'd love to marry you, Daniel.' She knelt down on the floor beside him, throwing her arms around him.

For her, knowing he was going to be there for her in sickness and in health, loving her and honouring her for ever, was an even greater gift than all the jewels in the world.

* * * * *

If you enjoyed this story,
check out these other great reads
from Karin Baine

Nurse's New Year with the Billionaire
Festive Fling with the Surgeon
Midwife's One-Night Baby Surprise
Highland Fling with Her Boss

All available now!

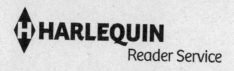
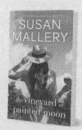 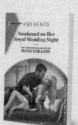 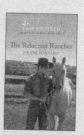 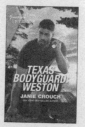